MW01673195

Motorcycle Smarts

Overcome Fear
Learn Control
Master Riding Well

Copyright and Disclaimers

Motorcycle Smarts: Overcome Fear, Learn Control, Master Riding Well

Copyright © 2021

All rights reserved. Except as permitted under the U.S. Copyright Act of 1976, no part of this publication may be reproduced, distributed, or transmitted in any form or by any means, or stored in a database or retrieval system, without the prior written permission of the publisher.

Disclaimer

While all attempts have been made to verify the information provided in this publication, neither the author nor the publisher assumes any responsibility for errors, omissions, or contrary interpretations of the subject matter herein. The views expressed are those of the author alone, and should not be taken as expert instruction or imperatives. The reader is responsible for his or her own actions.

Contents

Warning

Every time I suit up to ride, I weigh my options and evaluate my risks. As long as the pleasure of riding overshadows the additional exposure, I'll continue to throw a leg over and strap on my helmet.

When it doesn't, I'll stop riding.

The risks are real. Motorcycle crashes—often caused by negligent motorists—can cause serious injuries, even death.

In this book, I attempt to present accurate information that will ultimately make you a safer rider. But I'm human. My advice may not apply to every rider in every situation.

No book, including this one, can teach you how to ride a motorcycle proficiently. Please seek lessons from a licensed instructor.

Ride safely and at your own risk.

Foreword

The Author's Motorcycle Mentor

I once read that we each have a gene that controls how we relate to our environment in terms of our excitement level.

I knew a fellow once who needed to ride his motorcycle at insane speeds to feel a satisfying level of fun. My excitement gene isn't like that. It doesn't take much speed for me to be thrilled, whether in a car, on a bike, or snow skiing.

Maybe that makes me a conservative rider.

When David approached me in 2005 about helping him get into this amazing hobby, I took the same careful approach I did when riding. My primary concern for David was safety, but I also believe that riding safely is an outcome of knowledge and preparation.

At the time, I had ridden well over 100,000 miles without going down—unless we count the time in my driveway when I thought the side stand was out (it wasn't) and pushed the bike over.

I put out my hand to save my head and broke my wrist.

When David came to me for advice, his enthusiasm was something to behold. He was the perfect student, and I was glad to help him.

I wanted him to understand the basics (my favorite examples being countersteering and seeing) so he could safely ingrain good riding techniques and then begin to enjoy the feeling of freedom that comes from riding. I believe he reached that goal and more.

David truly understands motorcycles, and I am honored to have been his motorcycle mentor.

Introduction

THE TRUTH IS THIS. RIDING A MOTORCYCLE WELL IS PART SKILL, PART WILLING TO LEARN, PART UNDERSTANDING OF BASIC PHYSICS, AND PART GIVING A DAMN ABOUT YOUR SAFETY AND THE SAFETY OF THOSE AROUND YOU.

Two men spent a considerable amount of time mentoring me when I first started riding a motorcycle.

They nurtured my passion for learning how motorcycles work. I studied everything I could find, and I practiced everything I learned. The *Motorcycle Smarts* book series is my attempt to pay that forward.

I wrote this book because I couldn't find one like it when I started riding. Motorcycle magazine columns converted into books are hard to follow—while other motorcycling books tend to focus on the wrong topics. Even with my engineering background, reading 300-plus pages attempting to explain everything about motorcycling feels painful.

You don't have to know everything to ride well.

You don't need to know how to change a tire, replace a headlight, or understand that rake angle affects how quickly you can flick your bike in a turn. You don't need to understand how your engine works.

And you certainly don't need to understand gyroscopic precision.

On the other hand, there are topics that every rider should understand in order to REDUCE THEIR CHANCES OF CRASHING.

This book tackles *these* topics in seven main sections:

PART ONE explores a rarely talked about phenomenon that most riders experience called *rider fear*. What is it? Who has it? What can you do to make it go away? What should you do if it doesn't?

Rider fear is real, and it shouldn't be ignored.

PART TWO introduces the importance of *YOU*. You can't become a proficient rider if you don't take ownership of improving your riding skills. Learn with your head, first, then practice until you develop the muscle memory to perform the movement correctly.

YOU are the most important part of your riding safety.

PART THREE defines and explains *countersteering*. This is one of the most important, yet often misunderstood, topics in the motorcycling community. I'll explain why and hopefully convince you that countersteering is the single most important way you control your motorcycle. Once you master it, you'll be able to make your motorcycle go where you want it to go (instinctively) with small inputs to the handlebar.

PART FOUR explains *lowside* and *highside* crashes. What are they? What causes them? What can you do to avoid them? I've included illustrations of real crashes (captured on video) and break them down frame-by-frame so you can understand what's happening.

PART FIVE covers *braking, electronics,* and the *Hurt Report*. In this section, I'll unpack ABS (along with Traction Control) and tackle the myth that you should avoid using your front brake. We'll also look at the Hurt Report—the most comprehensive study of why riders crash.

The Hurt Report will change the way you ride. I promise.

PART SIX has a few closing thoughts and my personal challenge.

And finally, in the APPENDIX, I introduce my motorcycle mentors, give a sneak peek of my next book in the *Motorcycle Smarts* book series that documents my ride from Alabama to Alaska with my best friend, and share what listeners have said about the *Motorcycle Mentor Podcast*.

As a bonus, I've added several chapters on more lighthearted topics and sprinkled them throughout the book to give the reader a break.

My goal isn't for you to agree with everything I profess.

Some will say I'm over the top in certain areas—by nagging you to practice for every possible situation, and obsessing over ABS as though it solves all the world's problems. But others will say I'm too lax in other areas—by not preaching that you should wear a full face helmet.

What you wear on your head is your business.

Hold on Tight

I have to warn you. There's a lot of information packed into this book. Stick with me, though, because once you understand and incorporate this material, I honestly believe you'll be less likely to crash.

Am I saying you can reduce your risk to zero? NO!

Skilled riders crash and die every day when there was NOTHING they could have done to avoid it. But it is also true that under-skilled riders crash and die every day when there WAS something they could have done to avoid it.

In the end, I believe with all my heart that …

ALL RIDERS CAN CHANGE THEIR CHANCES OF CRASHING.

Who Should Read This Book?

This book isn't just for riders starting out.

This is the book I'd hand to someone who's been riding for decades and wants to reduce their risks of crashing. It's also the book I'd give to my son if he told me he wanted to learn how to ride.

Back in 2007, I invited my mentors to my house for an evening of motorcycle talk in my basement. After a few minutes of light conversation, I pulled out a stack of notes, looked them in the eyes, and said:

"Someday, I want to explain motorcycles my way."

THIS BOOK IS THAT VISION.

It took me more than ten years. I did everything I could to put it off. But I knew deep in my soul that I had to finish this book, so I did. If it helps just one rider, I've accomplished what I set out to do.

I want this book to change the way you think about motorcycling.

I want this book to change the way you ride.

You're in the right place, and I'm thrilled you're here.

Wait. There's one last thing I need to warn you about.

I call the thing I write about in this book a motorcycle and a bike.

I mostly blame my riding buddy (and friend) Mike for teaching me this. I found it strange the first hundred or so times he referred to his motorcycle as a bike. It wasn't long before I did the same.

My parents were right.
You <u>are</u> influenced by the people you hang out with.

Mastering the Art of Riding Well

If I didn't think I could measurably reduce my chances of being in a crash, I wouldn't ride. I believe you can reduce your chances too.
— DAVID MIXSON

MASTERING THE ART OF RIDING A MOTORCYCLE WELL is about learning how to ride the right way. It's about taking each ride seriously. It's about enjoying the experience and making good decisions based on the laws of physics.

It's about being confident you can avoid distracted drivers. It's about having a plan before you need a plan. It takes effort.

It's about understanding and overcoming rider fear, and having the head knowledge of how your motorcycle works so you can make it go where you want it to go. It's about understanding why riders crash.

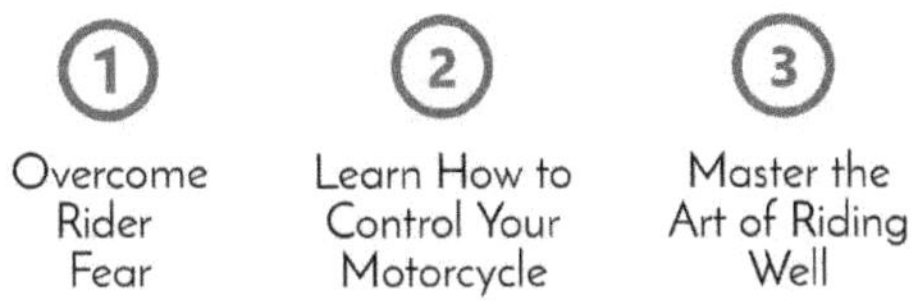
1
Overcome Rider Fear
2
Learn How to Control Your Motorcycle
3
Master the Art of Riding Well

Learning how to control your motorcycle should be your primary goal when you buy your first motorcycle, or your next goal if you've ridden for decades. *Control* is the skill that makes you less likely to be in an accident. It's the path to proficient riding.

Too many riders get bogged down trying to select the perfect bike and thinking that buying the right gear is the most important part of the journey. It's not. And it's the reason why I don't talk about these topics in this book—the first book in the *Motorcycle Smarts* series.

I'm not saying riding gear isn't important. I'm saying that you don't need to spend all your time selecting it. Instead, focus on overcoming rider fear and learning how to control your motorcycle.

Only then can you MASTER THE ART OF RIDING WELL.

A Fresh Approach

Every study on motorcycle crashes I've seen says the same thing:

Riders are making the same mistakes we did decades ago—even with mandatory training and plenty of books on the subject.

An NHTSA study in *2012* found that motorcyclists were 26 times more likely than car occupants to die in accidents (per mile traveled).[1] A similar NHTSA study in *2018* showed that riders are now 28 times more likely to die in motor vehicle traffic crashes.[2]

What we're doing to educate riders isn't working.

We need a fresh approach.

The *Motorcycle Smarts* book series is my attempt to do that.

The foundation of every book I've written on motorcycles begins with a core belief that every rider can change their chances of crashing.

My passion has never wavered, and I doubt it ever will.

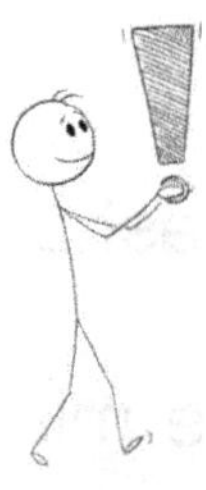

The real issue isn't that riders get banged up when they crash. That's a given.
It's that average riders crash by themselves way too often making the same mistakes riders did generations ago.

Average riders use their rear brake way too much, don't know what lowside crashes are (and what causes them), and say there's little they can do to keep from crashing—thinking, *when my time comes, it comes*.

Average riders make errors that account for half of all crashes, don't know how to react when a driver makes a mistake, and choose whether to wear a helmet based on whether their riding buddies wear one.

Average riders consider fashion over function way too often.

Average riders do the same things average riders did decades ago.

Don't fall into the trap of thinking the way to have riders crash less is to make them wear helmets. Helmets don't keep us from crashing.

I don't care what you wear or what you ride. I care that you understand how motorcycles work so you can master why they crash. Once you do this, you can avoid triggering some of the most common types of crashes—and maybe even outlive your riding buddies.

It's time for a fresh approach to explaining how motorcycles work and how they crash—so a wife won't be left without her husband, a husband without his wife, or a child without their parent.

Something's not working. We need a fresh approach.

Rider Fear Can be Pretty Persistent

Part One: Rider Fear

Overcoming rider fear is the first step.

This section wasn't in the original version of this book, but I knew something was missing, so I added it. Rider fear is real, it's paralyzing, and it shouldn't be ignored. If you're a seasoned rider and don't have rider fear, you might want to read through this section pretty fast. If you have severe anxiety when you ride (or merely think about riding), this section is for you.

ONE

Helmet Thoughts

Something magical happens when I put on a motorcycle helmet.

I see my life from a different viewpoint. I think of things to tell my wife and childhood stories to share with my kids. I mull over tasks I need to complete around the house and actions I need to take at work to be more effective. I ponder items to add to my bucket list.

And I feel thankful for the blessings in my life.

I'm pretty sure it's not the helmet that makes me think so clearly. Rather it's the intimacy of riding through Mother Nature.

Maybe it's the hum of the engine or the sound of wind rushing by.

Maybe it's the quiet peace of knowing I can't call someone—and that someone can't call me.

This magic doesn't happen on every ride, but it happens on some. And that's good enough. Sometimes, I wonder if I'm the only one who has these magical thoughts inside my helmet.

If that's the case, lucky me.

TWO

What Is Rider Fear?

When I pulled into traffic for the first time,
I nearly freaked out.
— David Mixson

In this section, I'll explain what I've learned for myself (and from others) about the topic I call *rider fear*.

I started my first website on motorcycles more than a decade ago. Without question, I've received more emails about rider fear than any other topic. I'll share some of these emails as we go along.

RIDER FEAR is the pit in your stomach when you think about riding a motorcycle. It's your heart racing when you venture out into traffic. It's the overwhelming sensation you're not in control.

Every rider defines it differently. Some describe it as an uncomfortable feeling, while others say it feels more like a panic attack.

Here's how one rider described rider fear:

"I have always wanted to ride a motorcycle. Six months ago I bought a used motorcycle a riding friend helped me pick out. She is a great rider and has encouraged me to fulfill my dreams of riding a motorcycle. I practiced in parking lots for the first few weeks and then took a training class. I really enjoyed the class and learned a lot. I passed the rider test on my first attempt. I was so excited. As long as I ride in parking lots and in my neighborhood, I feel fine. But just the thought of venturing out onto busy streets causes me to panic, and a fear comes over me like nothing I've experienced in my 44 years."

Here's how another rider described it:

"All my motorcycle friends have been riding for years and don't seem to understand the fear and lack of confidence I have in what I'm doing."

Do all riders experience rider fear? No. But based on the number of emails

I've received, most do—some to the point of doubting everything (including their decision to ride).

Here's how Cathy described it:

> *"I have so much fear it's a shame. When I see my motorcycle, fear comes over me. When I get on it, it's even worse. Please help me overcome this."*

My Personal Story

I vividly recall my first ride in traffic.

I had just purchased my first motorcycle, a bright red Honda VFR, and wanted to take it out for a spin. I borrowed a helmet and riding jacket from a friend and ventured out on my own.

Everything started out fine. I did a few laps in the parking lot of an apartment complex near my house, and from there I ventured out to a side street at a nearby shopping center.

I felt a little nervous but nothing too bad.

A short time later, I decided to venture out into traffic. I exited the shopping center and turned right onto Highway 72 heading west. My heart started racing. Cars were all around me. I felt anxious, awkward, and incredibly small. My mind became overwhelmed.

What if I dropped my motorcycle at a busy intersection?

What would it feel like if I crashed?

What would I do if someone came into my lane, or pulled out in front of me, or stopped abruptly?

Is this really a good idea?

Did I purchase the right motorcycle?

Am I selfish for wanting to ride, especially since this whole thing makes my family nervous?

Do I even enjoy riding?

And then I thought: If I die in an accident today, my motorcycle mentor (an avid reader) will certainly find out. The headline reads:

"Beginning Rider Crashes During First Ride in Traffic."

I rode a five-mile loop that afternoon, making only right-hand turns because left-hand turns seemed too hard. How could it be that such a short ride physically and mentally consumed me?

I felt under-skilled and vulnerable. When the ride was over, I took off my helmet and made this promise to myself.

If this fear doesn't go away, I will sell my motorcycle and stop riding.

RIDER FEAR IS REAL. IT'S FRIGHTENING. AND IT POKES ITS HEAD OUT WHENEVER IT WANTS.

Key Points

1. Rider fear is real. My email inbox proves it.

2. Rider fear can range from anxiety to debilitating panic.
3. I had never heard of rider fear before I experienced it for myself. That's why I think it's important we talk about it.

THREE

Who Has Rider Fear?

If you have at least some level of rider fear, you're probably normal.
— David Mixson

Now that we've defined rider fear, let's talk about who has it.

Rider fear isn't biased. Men and women can have rider fear, as can young riders and old riders, beginning riders and experienced riders.

Beginning riders, however, seem most likely to experience it. I estimate that well over half (maybe more) of all beginning riders experience a heightened level of fear and anxiety when they first start riding. While experienced riders can also encounter this same fear, it's usually less intense.

Here's what Betty wrote:

> *"I hate to admit this, but my motorcycle seems more like an enemy than a friend. I'm paralyzed with fear. I'm frustrated. Practicing in parking lots and my neighborhood isn't much fun. How do I get through this fear? Please help."*

Over the years, I've noticed a special group of riders that struggles with rider fear—riders who feel pressured to ride. Often it's a woman who's ridden as a passenger and decides she wants to ride on her own bike. When this happens, her husband does what any good husband should do. He encourages her.

Everything usually starts out fine. It's a logical (simple) step to go from passenger to rider, right? Not always.

Here's what Helen wrote:

"I have ridden as a passenger with my husband for almost 15 years. This past spring, I decided I wanted to ride my own bike. Almost immediately, a fear overcame me. Even after taking the MSF course twice (and passing both times), I still don't feel comfortable riding. I start dreading our rides the night before. My husband doesn't understand how I feel because he's been riding since he was a kid. He wants us to take a trip on our motorcycles this summer, but I don't want to. I hate myself for feeling this way. I don't want him to be disappointed. I feel stuck."

Helen wants to overcome her fear and please her husband.

But rider fear is telling her something different.

Why am I highlighting this group of riders?

Because Helen isn't the only one in this predicament who's contacted me, and because feeling pressured to ride can make you do things you probably shouldn't.

On the one hand, your body is telling you to stop riding. On the other hand, your spouse (or friend) is telling you to battle through your fear and not give up. This can be a dangerous combination.

Don't let others silence your inner voice.

Don't mistake encouragement for pressure.

Don't ride just because someone else wants you to.

It's wrong, and it's dangerous.

Key Points

1. Rider fear isn't biased. It likes all riders.
2. Beginning riders should expect rider fear.

3. Don’t ride just because someone else wants you to.

FOUR

How to Overcome Rider Fear

Rider fear is usually rooted in a lack of confidence in your riding skills.
— David Mixson

Now that you know what rider fear is and who usually has it, let's take a look at the best ways to overcome it.

When I first started riding, all my attention was focused on operating my motorcycle. I didn't have anything left to prepare for *what-if* scenarios, and I certainly didn't have the riding skills to avoid stupid driver mistakes.

My anxiety decreased as my skills improved.

It wasn't immediate, but it was steady. After every new experience (rain, cold, traffic, interstate), I became more confident in my abilities.

As the mechanics of operating my motorcycle became easier, I was able to devote more of my attention to riding defensively and enjoying the beauty of Mother Nature around me.

Making Rider Fear Go Away

For most, rider fear will disappear or become more manageable as your riding skills improve. But for some, rider fear will never go away.

In fact, it might even become more intense.

Unfortunately, there's no magic quick fix that will make rider fear vanish. But here are some things you can do that will usually help.

1. Overcome rider fear by learning how motorcycles work.

I strongly believe that all riders should learn the basics of how motorcycles work. Learn how motorcycles work (with your head first) and good things will usually follow.

Here's what Joe said:

> *"The MSF class was worth every dime and a lot of fun. However, two weeks after my class I went riding with some friends from work on a busy street. Making a wide right turn, I got tunnel vision on the median strip and went into it like a moth into a bug zapper. It was more embarrassing than anything, but all the talk during the MSF class about keeping your head up and pointed where you want to go suddenly made more sense."*

In this example, Joe fell into the trap of looking where he *didn't* want to go, instead of focusing on the path where he *did* want to go.

This is called *target fixation*, a subject I cover in more depth later. The important thing to note here is that *head knowledge* warns us of target fixation, something no amount of riding by itself could.

In my mind, you can't become a proficient rider without understanding the fundamentals of how motorcycles work. I wrote this book because I wanted to simplify (shorten) this process for riders.

It's the book I looked for (but couldn't find) when I started riding.

2. Overcome rider fear by learning control.

I firmly believe that rider fear is rooted in a *lack of confidence* in your ability to control your motorcycle. Will all rider fear magically go away once you master control? No. But learning how to make your bike do what you want it to will usually move you in the right direction.

The most important thing here is putting what you learn about motorcycles into practice. As an example, in a later chapter, you will learn that you should favor your front brake over your rear brake.

This is *head knowledge*.

Once you understand this, the next step is to use your front brake. Use the correct technique when you practice, and you'll instinctively use the correct technique when it matters the most.

3. Overcome rider fear by taking hands-on training.

One of the best ways to reduce rider fear is to take a hands-on training class. I address this topic in more depth in a later chapter.

But here, I'll make this point.

There's something really powerful about having a trained motorcycle instructor guide you in a one-on-one setting. If you have rider fear and aren't sure what to do next, take another training class.

Here's what Beth told me about hands-on training:

"I started riding in my 20s. My brothers and I learned by hitting the dirt trails and exploring. I eventually stopped riding, however, because of the fear I felt when riding in traffic. Now almost 45 years later, I got the bug again at 67, signed up for an MSF class, and passed with the help of an amazing teacher. The training showed me how to maneuver my bike and make good decisions. Without this class, the fear would have completely taken over again. Now I have [the head] knowledge of how to ride and a reasonable expectation of my limits."

4. Overcome rider fear by practicing.

Want to kick rider fear in the butt? Want to improve your riding skills? Want to MASTER THE ART OF RIDING YOUR MOTORCYCLE WELL?

Then you must practice your craft. I address this topic in more depth in a later chapter. But here, I'll make this point.

Practice in your driveway. Practice in your neighborhood. Practice in a vacant parking lot. Practice starting and stopping. Practice low-speed turns. Practice the things you learned in your hands-on training. Practice in all weather conditions.

Learn something new every time you ride.

I like Bill's approach:

> *"I'm a beginning rider at age 48, and I'm afraid. I'm taking it slow and practicing in parking lots at my own speed and comfort level. I'm less fearful after each practice session, and I try to attain a new goal during every ride. The more I ride, the more I understand what I need to work on to become a skilled and safe rider."*

Riding frequently is one of the best ways to improve your riding skills. My motorcycle mentor encouraged me to practice as often as I could, even if I only had a few minutes.

To this day, I look at every ride as an opportunity to learn something new. What did I do well? What do I need to work on next time?

5. Overcome rider fear by staying in your comfort zone.

My best advice to riders struggling with rider fear is to stay inside, or just slightly outside, your comfort zone. As your skills improve, slowly expand your comfort zone.

Once you master your driveway, head out into your neighborhood. Once you master your neighborhood, find simple roads with no traffic, and from there more difficult roads with traffic.

Here's how Robin did it:

"At 38 I asked myself why not. I've wanted to ride a motorcycle for most of my adult life. It was hard at first. I rode in parking lots—lots and lots of parking lots. Taking a rider course really propelled me, yet that first ride

on a real road had me trembling. I made so many mistakes that I questioned whether riding a motorcycle was right for me. I wondered if I was doing it out of stubbornness. I stuck with it and rode every chance I could. Before each ride, I would ask myself whether I was having a good day or bad and alter my route accordingly. I worked on specific skills during each ride and was amazed at how fast things improved. My confidence soared."

6. Overcome rider fear by constantly reevaluating your progress.

As you move through this journey, your riding skills should improve, and your rider fear should become less intense. Give yourself time and then reevaluate how you feel.

The most important thing to look for is steady progress.

Progress means you're on the right track.

7. Overcome rider fear by listening.

It's never a good idea to try to silence your rider fear. Instead, embrace it and listen to what it's telling you to do.

When is your rider fear most intense?

Do you dread riding or look forward to it?

Is someone encouraging you to ride?

Do you need to work on the mechanics of riding?

Would taking another hands-on training class help?

Listen to your body, and it will usually show you where you need to improve. In the next chapter, we'll talk about what you should do if your rider fear won't go away. But before we move forward, I want you to make the following commitment to yourself.

You are more than worth it.

"I [your name] will listen to what my body is telling me. I will let others encourage me, but I will not allow them to influence my decision to ride a motorcycle. I will take responsibility for my own actions. And in the end, if my fear doesn't go away, or at least become manageable, I will take this as a sign and stop riding."

Two months after my first ride in traffic, I reevaluated how I felt. The fear was less intense, and I still enjoyed riding. I was prepared to follow through on the promise I made to myself to stop riding.

And I still am.

Key Points

1. Rider fear is almost always rooted in a lack of confidence.
2. Learning how motorcycles work is the best first step in learning how

to control your motorcycle—and directly on the path to reducing rider fear.

3. Listen to what your body is telling you. It's usually right.

FIVE

My Rider Fear Isn't Going Away

Sometimes rider fear can be pretty stubborn.
— David Mixson

Let's assume you've followed the process I outlined in the last chapter, but your rider fear hasn't gone away as fast as you'd like.

In this situation, you have two options. The best course of action for most is to push through it until you master your craft. But for others, the best path forward is to stop riding.

Some are shocked when I say this. Others are relieved.

I hesitate giving specific advice to riders who can't shake rider fear. On the one hand, I believe that fear robs us of our dreams and it needs to be overcome and destroyed, regardless. I pushed through rider fear and tons of other riders have too.

Here's a rider who persevered:

> *"I started riding when I was 40. The third time I had my motorcycle on the road I went off the edge on a bad bend, rode down a ditch, came back on the road, and the bike flipped end over end with me still on it. Got lots of road rash and stitches in my elbow. I tried to ride it again after it was repaired, but I was shaky and scared. I sold the bike and rode with my husband. Fast forward seven years. Feeling envious when my neighbor got a Harley, I bought her Honda Rebel. This time I did the smart thing and took the MSF safety class. I quickly realized how much I didn't*

know. I failed the class because I was still gun-shy and the instructors said I needed more seat time. I rode around and around the back streets of my neighborhood mastering the skills of starting, stopping, and using the clutch. Then I retook the class and passed! My husband bought me a new Sportster for Christmas. That was 13 years ago. I'm on my second Sportster now. I think the class gave me the skills I needed, and practice gave me the confidence."

Best-selling author Michael Hyatt wrote, "Discomfort is a catalyst for growth. There's no better way to grow in any area of your life than to consistently put yourself in uncomfortable situations."

He's right. Riders who overcome rider fear should celebrate.

BUT WAIT ... Rider fear can also be a friend that saves your life!

Fear is natural, instinctive, and unbiased. Fear is your body's way of telling you it's uncomfortable, out of balance, and in danger.

Fear can be a wonderful thing. It can show you where you need to improve. It can nudge you to take action. It should never be ignored.

Best-selling author Steven Pressfield wrote, "If you are paralyzed with fear, it's a good sign. It shows you what you have to do."

Here's a rider who listened:

> *"I have been struggling to feel comfortable riding a motorcycle for several years. After I received your kind email response, I decided that my soul (as you called it) was telling me to stop riding. Last month I sold my motorcycle. I feel so much better! I am so proud of my decision to stop riding."*

Now What?

Now that we've determined that fear can be good *and* bad, each of us has to determine what we do with it.

Do we stop riding when we have rider fear?

Do we try to overcome it?

Do we put our head down and ignore it?

Here's how Christopher plans on handling it:

"I rode motorcycles off-road as a kid. My dad always rode a Harley. Unfortunately, a drunk driver murdered my father while he was on his bike. I bought a new Harley for myself later that same year to join him for rides (like he always wanted). Long story short, I'm 44 now, and it's been ten years. I still have my 2003 Harley, but every time I get ready to ride I find some reason or sign not to. My nerves have driven me crazy. I feel bad, but I can't give up."

If I were Christopher, I would probably stop riding. But I'm not. Christopher is the only one who can make that decision.

In the end, you're the only one who can decide what to do next. Only you can determine if riding fulfills your dreams, fulfills someone else's dreams, or somehow rights a wrong.

When I had rider fear, I was looking for consistent improvements. I expected to have less fear this week than I did last week. I expected my riding skills to improve. I expected the mechanics of operating my motorcycle to become easier.

All this happened, so I kept riding.

My Best Advice

If you're experiencing the same intensity of rider fear after months of consistent riding, then I want you to ask yourself this simple question:

Do you really want to continue riding a motorcycle?

If you don't, take a deep breath and smile. I give you permission to stop riding. Your soul is telling you to stop, so stop.

It's not the end of the world. I promise.

Key Points

1. Consistent improvement signals you're on the right track.
2. Don't ride just because someone else wants you to.
3. There's no shame in choosing a different hobby.

SIX

Final Thoughts on Rider Fear

How can something so terrifying be so enticing?
— David Mixson

It's been more than a decade since I conquered rider fear, *or did I?*

To this day, before I put on my helmet, I pause, take a deep breath, and ask myself if I really want to do this.

Is my mind clear?

Do I feel steady and sure?

Is the reward worth the risk?

Fear can be a great motivator and guide. Fear isn't the enemy; it's our friend. Fear is how our unconscious mind steers our conscious mind. Fear is how our body prepares for peak performance. FEAR IS AMAZING!

If you're struggling with rider fear, I believe that the best path forward is for you to lean into your fear and listen to what it's telling you.

Rider fear is part of your journey.

It's how your soul tells your body it needs to improve.

Rider fear keeps you from doing things your muscles don't know how to do. It's a meter that registers progress. Rider fear is so beneficial that I feel sorry for riders who've never experienced it.

Ralph explains it this way:

"I rode motorcycles in my 20s and 30s then stopped. I started back when I turned 52. The first thing I did was take the MSF course at the local community college as a refresher.

There's always a bit of nervousness when the kickstand goes up, but for me, nervousness combined with awareness leads to heightened alertness. My grandfather owned a small plane for years but sold it when he stopped having that small butterfly knot in his belly at take-off. He thought he was becoming too confident in his abilities. He always said, 'There are old pilots and bold pilots, but no old, bold pilots.' Maybe a motorcyclist is just a two-dimensional aviator. Becoming complacent and over-confident could place you at the Pearly Gates ahead of schedule."

Ralph is right. Having at least some rider fear is probably a good thing. Don't look for rider fear to go away completely but to become more manageable as your riding skills improve.

Once you learn how to control your motorcycle, riding will seem easier. You'll be able to notice the beauty around you

—the intoxicating fragrances of spring and the cool crispness of fall.

Hal Elrod, author of *The Miracle Morning*, said:

> *"Everything is difficult before it's easy. Every new experience is uncomfortable before it's comfortable. The more you practice [your craft] the more natural and normal it will feel."*

Scuba diving is hard before it's easy.
Playing the piano is hard before it's easy.
Riding a motorcycle is HARD before it's easy.

For most riders, there's a good chance you'll look back on rider fear as a thing of the past, an obstacle you overcame, a feeling that made you get serious about learning how to control your bike. But for others, it will be a persistent guerrilla that destroys your dream of riding.

Either way, rider fear served a valuable purpose.

In the end, when your inner voice can't be silenced, it's probably time to follow her advice. If there's one thing I want you to take away from this book, it's this.

IT'S OKAY TO STOP RIDING A MOTORCYCLE.

My first ride in traffic changed the way I rode.

Rider fear showed me what I had to do to become a better rider.

Rider fear signaled when I was making progress and when I wasn't.

Rider fear probably saved my life.

And it can save yours too.

Key Points

1. Rider fear isn't the enemy. It's your friend.

2. Riding a motorcycle is difficult before it's easy.
3. When rider fear can't be calmed, it's probably time to follow her advice and choose a different hobby.

You <u>Can</u> Change Your Chances of Crashing

Part Two: All About You

Riding a motorcycle well begins with YOU.

In this section, we'll talk about taking ownership of your riding safety, practicing the correct way, and developing muscle memory. Nothing great happens if you don't get this part right. This section is the foundation for the how-to material that follows.

SEVEN

An Old Country Store

One of the most enjoyable parts of riding is exploring places I've never been. It's simple to do. I head north (or south or east or west) from my house and turn onto roads I've never traveled.

I'm always amazed at how things can change such a short distance from my congested life. City streets and highways turn into country roads. Walmart Super Centers disappear—and country stores appear.

When I was a kid, there was a country store about a mile from my grandparent's farm. My sister and I used to walk there to buy candy.

Banana taffy was my favorite.

The walk was always worth it, even in the blistering southern heat. With a handful of change, we could leave with a pocketful of candy that would last us all day.

The pieces seemed bigger back then.

I didn't realize old country stores still existed until I purchased a motorcycle. I'm thrilled they still do.

Find one for yourself and see what I mean. It's like stepping back in time. Imagine what it must have felt like to buy a piece of candy for a penny or a candy bar for a nickel.

That's what I do.

A few of the country stores I've discovered look like they haven't changed much in the last 50 years. Those are my favorites. There is truly something magical about getting away from the modernness of our normal surroundings to a place that reminds us of our past.

The next time you find an old country store—stop and enjoy.

EIGHT

Take Ownership of Your Safety

Motorcycle safety is a choice.
— David Mixson

Now that we've listened to what rider fear had to say, let's talk about the most important component of becoming a better rider. YOU.

It's hard for me to understand this, but some riders don't think they can reduce their chances of crashing. Instead of taking responsibility for riding better *offensively* (by improving their riding skills) and *defensively* (by looking out for the other guy), they place their faith in mathematical statistics and believe:

"When my time comes, it comes."

Don't fall into the trap of thinking this way!

Here are six things you can do to ride more safely.

1. Taking ownership of your riding safety is about believing you can reduce your risk of crashing.

In large part, the purpose of this book is to show the MOTORCYCLING COMMUNITY THEY CAN CHANGE THEIR CHANCES OF CRASHING.

Making this affirmation is the most important step in your journey to MASTERING THE ART OF RIDING WELL. This is because there is zero motivation to take action if you don't believe your actions will influence the outcome.

I realize that I'll have to convince some of you.

I'll do this by breaking down how motorcycles work, by explaining how to avoid certain types of crashes caused by rider error, by highlighting what the Hurt Report teaches us about why riders crash, and by deciphering motorcycle electronic systems that can virtually eliminate certain types of crashes.

2. Taking Ownership of Your Riding Safety Is About

UNDERSTANDING HOW TO CONTROL YOUR MOTORCYCLE.

And the foundation for understanding how to control your motorcycle is *head knowledge*. Understand how countersteering works so you can use it to make your motorcycle go where you want it to go. Understand lowside and highside crashes (and what causes them) so you can avoid them. Understand how to effectively use your brakes so you can stop faster.

3. TAKING OWNERSHIP OF YOUR RIDING SAFETY IS ABOUT IMPROVING YOUR DEFENSIVE RIDING SKILLS.

I've avoided crashing on numerous occasions by anticipating what motorists might do. Like the time I was riding on I-65 heading north toward Nashville, Tennessee. I was in the right lane, and a motorist in the left lane shot across in front of me to make the exit ramp.

I had just slowed down so I wasn't beside him, just in case.

Anticipate where drivers might want to go, and be somewhere else.

4. Taking ownership of your riding safety is about improving your offensive riding skills.

One of the best ways to do this is to take a hands-on training class. No book (including this one), training video, or Internet search can substitute for hands-on instruction.

Rider coaches are worth their weight in gold. Let them help you. More on how to get the most out of your training in the next chapter.

5. Taking ownership of your riding safety is about constantly improving.

The best riders I know say they *never stop learning*. Before and after every ride, think about what you need to work on.

Better yet, write your thoughts in a journal so you can monitor your progress.

6. Taking ownership of your riding safety is about having the right mindset.

It's about engaging in the idea that you can always do more to get better. It's about staying interested long enough to read this book all the way through. It's about caring about your loved ones enough to take this stuff seriously. Here's the honest truth.

If you want to be a better-than-average rider you have to THINK DIFFERENTLY THAN AVERAGE RIDERS. You need a different MINDSET.

Riding a motorcycle is hard. Riding a motorcycle proficiently is harder. Reading this book is a wonderful first move toward …

MASTERING THE ART OF RIDING WELL.

Congratulations. You're on the right track.

Key Points

1. YOU are responsible for your riding safety.
2. Work to improve your offensive and defensive riding skills.
3. Mindset is a catalyst that makes average riders great.

NINE

Take Hands-On Training

We've already touched on the importance of taking hands-on training. In this chapter, we'll expand on the topic and talk about how you can get the most out of your training.

Most states require that riders complete a hands-on training class as part of their motorcycle license endorsement. When I started riding again at forty, I still had my motorcycle endorsement from when I was fifteen. I took a hands-on training class anyway.

To get the most out of your training, make sure to select a program geared toward your riding level. Inexperienced riders should look for classes focused on helping beginning riders learn the basics. Experienced riders should look for classes focused on helping seasoned riders improve their riding skills.

So Many Options

The Motorcycle Safety Foundation (MSF) offers classes for riders at different skill levels. Their Basic Rider Course (BRC) is for beginner riders. If you don't have a motorcycle, that's not a problem.

The BRC supplies the bike and helmet.

The course consists of both classroom and hands-on instruction. The hands-on portion is conducted in a closed-off parking lot.

MSF isn't your only option. Since you are working toward your motorcycle license endorsement, it's a good idea to check with your Department of Motor

Vehicles (DMV) for a list of approved courses.

Training Day Tips

To get the most out of your training, take it seriously.

Think of it this way. You could learn something during class that saves your life.

Get a good night's sleep.

Show up early.

Bring the right gear to be comfortable.

I took my first hands-on course in the middle of winter. I wasn't as prepared as I should have been and struggled to stay warm. Don't make the same mistake. If it's cold, dress in layers and bring plenty of gear to stay warm. Carry gloves.

Trust me. It's hard to ride if you can't feel your fingers.

Check the course guidelines. Most require long sleeves and pants. If it's hot outside, a mesh riding jacket works great. If you don't have one, it's probably okay to improvise.

Just check first because the guidelines change.

Who Knew?

I took my first hands-on training class with a friend—the same friend I rode to Alaska with a decade later. Our instructor was great.

I now understand some of the things he was trying to get us to understand (like countersteering). I wish I could have read this book before taking the training.

He would have made more sense.

Key Points

1. Take hands-on motorcycle training seriously.
2. Read the course materials ahead of time if possible.
3. Ask questions during the class. Most rider coaches become rider

coaches because they want to help others.

TEN

Practice Everything

The more I practice, the luckier I get.
— Arnold Palmer

I've worked as an engineer at NASA for more than 30 years.

For nearly a decade of that time, I worked in the payload operations area conducting science experiments during Space Shuttle flights.

One of the most valuable lessons I took away from this experience is that the best way to learn how to perform a task well is to practice that task over and over again.

Before the Space Shuttle ever took off, we spent hundreds of hours in ground-simulations practicing for every imaginable scenario.

We practiced as if the experiments worked correctly.

We practiced workarounds in case they didn't.

By the time we made it to flight, the ground controllers—working with the astronauts onboard—knew how to handle most anything.

The actual missions were always easier.

Becoming proficient at riding a motorcycle is no different than becoming proficient at operating experiments in space. They both require PREPARATION and PRACTICE.

David L. Hough, author of *Proficient Motorcycling*, wrote."The moral of the story is that we must constantly practice the right skills if we expect to use them in a pinch."

How will you know how to make an emergency stop if you don't practice? How will you know how to use countersteering to avoid an object in the road if you don't practice? How will you become proficient at putting your bike on the center stand if you don't practice?

You won't.

Practice ... Practice ... Practice

Practice starting and stopping. Practice riding in the cold and the heat. Practice riding on curvy roads and straight roads, in groups and solo. Practice riding in traffic. Practice riding in the rain.

Practice riding in traffic when it's raining.

Practice using your brakes. Practice using countersteering to dodge objects in your path (more on this later). Practice staying calm when someone around you does something stupid.

Practice develops muscle memory (more on this later) and builds confidence. Practice is the foundation that makes you a better rider.

Practice the Correct Way

Before we leave the topic of practicing, I'll make this point. Practice is of little value unless you use the correct techniques while you practice.

My motorcycle mentor, Fred, insisted that I practice the right way, even when I was just riding around in my driveway.

"David, use the correct braking techniques in your neighborhood because that's what you'll instinctively use in a panic situation."

He was right.

A tennis player who swings with incorrect form while practicing will never become a great player, regardless of how much he practices.

Likewise, someone who rides a motorcycle with poor techniques while practicing will never become a proficient rider, regardless of how many hours he practices.

Take the stuff you learn in this book (and hands-on training) and practice the correct way in every situation—because that's how you'll do it when it matters.

Key Points

1. Practice makes perfect. Your parents were right.
2. Practice the big things and the little things.
3. Practice is the excuse you use to ride on the weekend. "Honey, I need to practice when it's sunny and in the 70s."

ELEVEN

Develop Muscle Memory

The trouble is very few of us can out-think our habits. In an emergency, we will do whatever we have been in the habit of doing, then think about it after the fact.

— David L. Hough, *Proficient Motorcycling*

Now that we've taken ownership of our riding safety and know to practice the correct way, let's talk about what we want to happen next.

When your muscles perform a sequence of movements over and over again, the activity naturally becomes easier. In effect, your muscles memorize how to perform the motions. This is called *muscle memory*.

The Oxford Dictionary defines muscle memory as:

"The ability to reproduce a particular movement without conscious thought, acquired as a result of frequent repetition of that movement."

A simple example of muscle memory is typing.

When I first started typing, I had to think about where each letter was located. Over time with lots of practice, my fingers (with the help of my brain) learned where each letter was located. Now, I don't think about moving my fingers to the correct keys. It just sort of happens.

Typing is now a part of my muscle memory.

A more complex example of muscle memory is throwing a baseball.

My son, Drew, took pitching lessons for years. Until then, I had no idea so many body parts have to move in sequence for a baseball to fly over home plate. Both arms and legs (along with head, hips, and back) must make precise movements at specific times during the motion for the ball to travel to the desired spot.

Drew looked awkward at first, and the ball went all over the place.

After every pitch, the coach told him what he needed to fix. "Push your gloved hand out sooner and extend your throwing arm earlier."

Once Drew understood what the coach wanted (head knowledge), he practiced the complex sequence of motions over and over until his brain made it a part of his muscle memory.

Spiking a Volleyball

It was the same for my daughter, Maddie, when she played volleyball.

Just like pitching, spiking a volleyball requires a complex sequence of motions performed at the exact right time.

Maddie looked awkward at first but worked hard to improve. First, by learning how to complete the motions (head knowledge), and then by practicing the correct way over and over again until it became a part of her muscle memory.

Over time, she no longer had to think about where to position her body. It all became automatic. With the help of muscle memory, she practiced her way to a college volleyball scholarship.

We use muscle memory every day.

Do you think about what your hands and feet should do when you drive? This is muscle memory. Do you consciously think about how to walk? This is muscle memory. Can you ride a bicycle even though you haven't ridden one in years? This is muscle memory.

Nobody Said This Was Easy

Operating a motorcycle is no different. Both arms and legs have to do stuff at the precise moment for it to go where you want it to go. Your muscles won't know how to do this at first—and your conscious brain will have to work extra hard.

But as you practice, the mechanics of riding will become a part of your muscle memory. Riding will seem easier—more automatic like typing or pitching or spiking. This is what you want.

Muscle memory is your reward for relentless practice.

It Gets Better

Here's the powerful part of all of this. Once the mechanics of operating a motorcycle become a part of your muscle memory, your *conscious* brain can focus on *defensive* riding skills (like looking for distracted drivers, noticing obstacles in the road, and finding the best lane position in traffic), and on *offensive* riding skills (like working on countersteering, using correct braking techniques, and looking where you want to go).

Muscle memory is why we practice.

Muscle memory makes us better riders.

> Muscle memory frees our mind to focus on things other than the MECHANICS OF OPERATING OUR MOTORCYCLE.

When I first started riding, I had to think about operating the clutch and shifting gears. I had to think about rolling off the throttle onto the front brake. I had to concentrate on looking deep into each turn.

After tons of practice, I don't have to think much about shifting gears or operating the clutch. It just sort of happens. The mechanics of operating a motorcycle is part of my muscle memory.

Now, I can think more clearly and focus on the beauty around me.

I can notice distracted drivers.

I can resist target fixation.

I can avoid the blind spot of the guy next to me.

This is the reason we should all strive for muscle memory.

Typing Class in High School

Before we close this chapter, let's take a step back and relook at the typing example mentioned earlier. I learned how to type in a business machines class back in high school. Every Friday afternoon my teacher gave us a speed test to see how many words we could type per minute.

At first, I was the slowest typist in the class because I did what the teacher asked us to do. "Class, type without looking at your keys."

I questioned my methodology after scoring so low on the first few speed tests. I could tell my friends were looking down at the keys.

It felt like they were cheating.

But I kept doing what the teacher told us to do because I figured she knew what she was talking about. It wasn't until several years later that I thought I knew more than adults my parents' age.

Guess What Happened?

My teacher wanted us to type without looking down at the keys when we practiced so we would develop the muscle memory to—drum roll please—type without looking at the keys.

Slowly but surely, my muscles learned where the keys were located and my speed steadily improved. It wasn't long before I could type more words per minute than anyone in the class. Why? Because I practiced the correct way until it became a part of my muscle memory.

To this day, I'm benefitting from the typing class I took back in high school. I typed most of this book without looking at the keys.

The only word that slowed me down—*motorcycle*.

Key Points

1. Muscle memory is our reward for disciplined practice.
2. Use proper techniques when you practice because that's the way your muscles will commit the task to memory.
3. As the mechanics of operating a motorcycle become easier, work on improving other aspects of your riding.

Countersteering Puts You in Control

Part Three: Countersteering

Countersteering is a wonderful thing.

It probably took me longer to understand countersteering than most. For some reason, my body didn't believe it could really be like this.

TWELVE

How My Motorcycle Changed Me

Riding a motorcycle has changed the way I look at my life.

I notice the beauty around me more purposefully.

I anticipate the warmth of spring and the coolness of fall.

I appreciate great riding days, even when I can't ride.

I've coined a phrase in my family that describes these near-perfect days. I call them *Top Ten Days*. You know the ones I'm talking about: blue skies, low humidity, and mild temperatures.

They usually show up in the spring and fall, but sometimes they make an appearance when you least expect them.

These are the most special.

We had a *Top Ten Day* last December. It was unseasonably warm, and my family was able to do something we had never done before. We ate outside at my wife's favorite restaurant on her birthday.

"Kids, this is a *Top Ten Day*," I said.

We all smiled and appreciated the moment—in large part because we paused long enough to notice.

I don't put a limit on the number of *Top Ten Days* I proclaim in a given year. Instead, I give thanks as often as possible.

It's a way to appreciate the beauty around me.

When you own a motorcycle, you'll see nature through a different lens. You'll no longer take for granted a clear blue sky framed with cotton-white clouds. *Top Ten Days* will call out to be enjoyed, whether on two wheels or not.

Riding a motorcycle changed me. It will change you too.

THIRTEEN

Before We Begin

He who loves practice without theory is like the sailor who boards a ship without a rudder and compass and never knows where he may cast.

— Leonardo da Vinci

If I had a weekend to talk to you about riding a motorcycle more proficiently, I'd focus on the information in the next few sections. THIS IS THE MATERIAL I PASSIONATELY BELIEVE EVERY RIDER SHOULD UNDERSTAND.

If you're an experienced rider and don't understand countersteering and lowside crashes, and have never heard of the Hurt Report, you're not alone. For many riders, these concepts have been missed along the way. Not because instructors don't understand them or think they're important, and not because the concepts are hard to understand.

Unfortunately, these topics are often buried in editorial-type magazine columns or insufficiently explained in motorcycle books.

As an example, just last week I picked up a mega book on motorcycling at a local bookstore. It had exactly one tiny paragraph on the entire topic of lowside crashes.

That's simply not enough space to explain what these crashes are—and more importantly—how you can avoid them. In comparison, the same mega book had an entire section on how to get the most out of your first Sturgis rally.

None of the material I'm about to present is unique. I didn't figure out something new that's never been figured out before. I'm just going deeper on certain subjects, the ones I believe are the most important, and with more gusto than other books.

I do this at the expense of NOT writing about other topics.

I'll leave the discussion of how to select riding gear and how to get the most out of your first motorcycle rally to other authors—for now.

Heads Up ...

Some of this material might seem overwhelming at first, but I break everything down in a non-engineering way—the way I learn best.

It's not important that you fully understand how countersteering works. It's important that you understand how to use countersteering to make your motorcycle go where you want it to go.

It's not important that you understand the physics of a lowside crash. It's important that you understand what triggers most lowside crashes so you can avoid them.

The main purpose of this book is to show you how you can CHANGE YOUR CHANCES OF CRASHING.
I do the bulk of the heavy lifting in the next three sections.

THIS IS THE STUFF THAT COULD SAVE YOUR LIFE.

FOURTEEN

Countersteering

It's hard to imagine that so many so-called "experienced" riders either fail to understand the importance of countersteering or fail to recognize that countersteering is how a motorcycle really turns.

— Ken Condon, *Riding in the Zone*

Now that we've learned the importance of practicing the correct way, let's talk about how we control our motorcycle using *countersteering*.

A textbook review of countersteering would require a discussion of a phenomenon known as gyroscopic precession. While this might be interesting to some, it's not important to understand the physics.

It's important to understand how countersteering gives us control.

My simplified but just as accurate definition of countersteering … the PHYSICS OF HOW YOU TURN your MOTORCYCLE.

If you've taken a hands-on training course or read a motorcycle skills book, you've heard the phrase "push right to go right" and "push left to go left." This is countersteering. This is how you control your bike.

See Figure 14-1 (below).

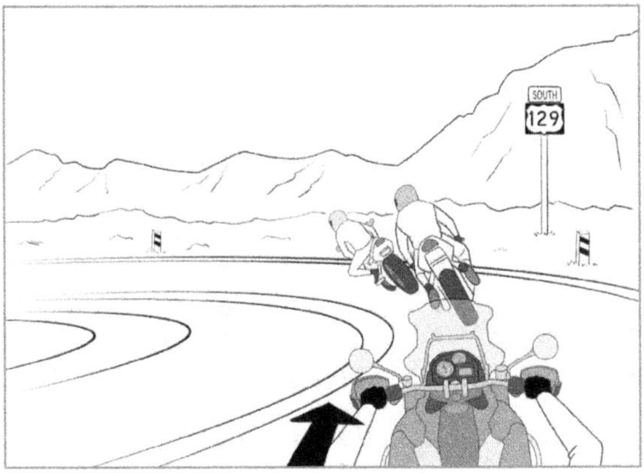

Figure 14-1 Countersteering (Push on Left Handlebar to Lean Left)

Sound Backwards?

You have probably noticed that countersteering is counterintuitive and *backward*. Pushing on the left handlebar is the same as turning (steering) the handlebar to the right. That's right, to initiate a turn you actually turn the handlebar in the *opposite* direction you want to go.

Let me say this again because I know it's hard to believe.

When you want to lean your motorcycle to the *left* (and turn left), you actually turn the handlebar to the *right* (which is the same input as pushing on the left handlebar).

This is true whether you realize it or not.

Isn't that amazing?

The motorcycle instructor gods of the past got it right when they crafted the slogan "push left to go left." They could have also said "turn right to go left," which is painfully confusing but equally correct.

If any of this sounds confusing, I understand. I struggled to make the mental connection of countersteering when I first started riding.

During my first MSF class, the instructor spent a great deal of time trying to get us to understand countersteering (with our head) and feel countersteering (with our body).

To do this, the instructor placed cones in a curve.

Then he had us ride around the curve faster and faster to force us to use countersteering to make the motorcycle turn in a tighter circle. The only way we could make the turn riding that fast was to push on the inside handlebar with purpose.

Over and over, the instructor called out, "Go faster. Make the bike lean more by pushing on the inside handlebar."

Countersteering didn't feel natural to me that day. My head didn't understand countersteering, and my body never made the connection. It wasn't until months later that countersteering made sense.

QUICK TIP: It's probably worth noting that countersteering doesn't start working until your wheels are rolling over a certain speed. There's passionate debate about the exact speed countersteering takes over. Some say countersteering starts working at about 15 mph. I say if your feet are comfortably up on the pegs, it's probably safe to assume that countersteering is at work.

Understanding Countersteering

Why do you need to understand countersteering with your head if you are using it already? You need to understand countersteering with your head so you can make your motorcycle go where you want it to go in every situation.

Countersteering is how you do normal turns.

Countersteering is how you dodge an object in the road.

It's what you use to make delicate adjustments in a sweeping turn. It's how you tighten a turn when you're running wide in a curve on a mountain pass where death is a real possibility if you run off the road.

Countersteering is powerful, but it doesn't require much input. An 80-pound woman can make an 800-pound Goldwing lean instantly.

Curves are easier once you master countersteering.

Push on your right handlebar gently to make your motorcycle lean (turn) to the right. Push on your left handlebar gently to make it lean (turn) to the left. If you need to tighten your turn radius, simply push a little more on the inside handlebar, and your bike will lean more.

Feeling Countersteering for Yourself

Once you understand countersteering with your head, it's time to feel it. In a vacant parking lot, find a spot on the pavement and practice swerving around it like it was an object in the road.

NOTE: If you can't find a spot, make your own by pouring a small amount of water on the pavement to darken it.

Approach the spot and swerve around it. Push right, push left, push right—will get you around the object to the right. Push left, push right, push left—will get you around the object to the left.

Here's another exercise.

In a vacant parking lot, come up to about 20 mph and take your left hand off the handlebar. Next, use only your throttle hand to make the motorcycle turn. Notice how it leans to the right when you push on the handlebar with your right hand, and leans to the left when you pull back on the right handlebar?

Feel it? You are turning the handlebar in the opposite direction.

Hence the term COUNTERsteering.

Keep Working

Don't stop until you make the mental connection of countersteering. Don't stop until it becomes a part of your muscle memory. Only then will you be able to use it to make your motorcycle go where you want it to go during the stress of an emergency.

Don't get frustrated. Mastering countersteering will take time. It certainly did for me. Be patient. Let your head and muscles put it all together over time.

It wasn't until I made the connection of how countersteering works that I felt confident riding and confident that I could make my motorcycle go where I wanted it to go.

COUNTERSTEERING IS THE PHYSICS THAT PUTS YOU IN CONTROL OF YOUR MOTORCYCLE.

Key Points

1. Learn how to use countersteering with your head, first.
2. Experiment with countersteering in a vacant parking lot. Keep practicing until you think to yourself, “I feel it!”
3. Countersteering puts you in control of your motorcycle.

FIFTEEN

Body Steering

Before we continue, it's probably worth noting that some riders don't believe countersteering is how you control your motorcycle.

Instead, they believe you lean (turn) your bike by *body steering*.

Shift your weight to the left to lean (turn) left.

Shift your weight to the right to lean (turn) right.

Keith Code, rider coach at the California Superbike School, got so tired of hearing naysayers rant that countersteering doesn't work that he modified a motorcycle to prove it does.

He calls it his *No B.S. Machine*.

Code's modified motorcycle has two sets of handlebars, the regular one from the factory and a second stationary set he added that doesn't rotate with the front forks.

Here's what Code found:

> *"At this writing, we have run nearly 100 riders of all experience levels on this double-barred bike. It has made believers out of every single one in the actuality of countersteering, of course. Even at speeds of no more than 20 to 35 mph, no matter how much you tug or push or pull or jump around on the bike, the best we saw was that the bike wiggled and became somewhat unstable. Did it turn? Not really. Would it turn at higher speeds? Absolutely not. Could you avoid something in your path? No way. Could anyone quick-turn the bike? Hopeless!"*[1]

The conclusion: Body Steering is a BIG FAT MYTH.

Key Points

1. Code's *No B.S. Machine* proves body steering is a myth.
2. Countersteering is how you make your motorcycle turn.

SIXTEEN

Tightening a Turn

Countersteering will save your life.
— KEN CONDON, *RIDING IN THE ZONE*

Why have I devoted an entire section in this book to the topic of countersteering? Because countersteering isn't just the way you control your motorcycle under normal conditions, it's how you control your motorcycle to avoid a crash.

Let's look at a common single-vehicle crash scenario.

Suppose you're on an interstate exit ramp around a curve sweeping to the right and have misjudged your speed. You're going wide toward the outside concrete barrier.

In this situation, you need to act quickly:

(1) look where you want to go deep in the curve,

(2) push on the inside handlebar to tighten your turn, and

(3) trust your tires to carry you through.

Believe me. This won't feel natural. The first time I did this, I was certain my tires would lose traction, but they didn't. I safely exited the turn and silently thanked my motorcycle mentor for teaching me to use countersteering and trust my tires.

The Way I Look at YouTube

FULL DISCLOSURE: I've never (knowingly) watched a video on YouTube that showed a rider being seriously injured or killed. That does me no good, and I think it's disrespectful to the rider and his family.

But YouTube can be a great tool if used properly—because there's usually a lesson buried in every motorcycle crash.

You've seen the videos, right?

Rider enters a curve and drifts wide off the road and crashes.

In most of the videos I've seen in this scenario, the rider's motorcycle wasn't leaned over very far, indicating the bike had more turning potential.

See Figure 16-1 (below).

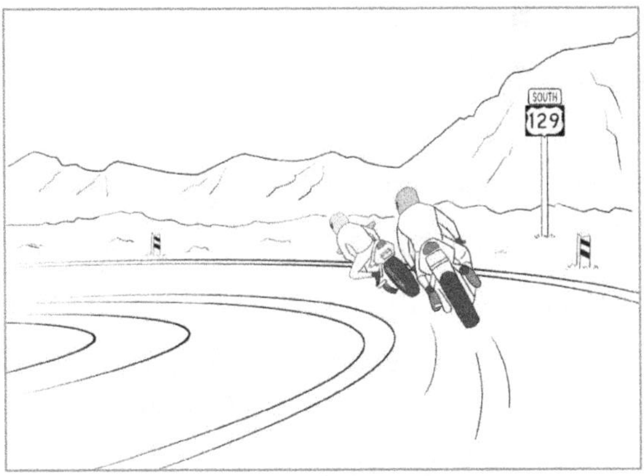

Figure 16-1 Countersteering to Tighten Turn (Push on Left Handlebar to Tighten Turn)

I can't help but wonder how many of these single-vehicle accidents could have been avoided if the rider had used countersteering and trusted his tires to tighten the turn?

Now you know why I'm so adamant that all riders UNDERSTAND COUNTERSTEERING with their HEAD.

Three Steps: Every—Single—Time

When you watch a wide-turn crash on YouTube, think about what the rider did incorrectly to be in that position.

Did he enter the curve too fast?

Did he enter on the wrong line?

Did he start his turn too early?

Regardless of his mistake, the solution is always the same: (1) look where you want to go, (2) push on the inside handlebar to tighten the turn, and (3) trust your tires.

Key Points

1. Motorcycle tires are amazingly sticky. When you get in a bind, give them a chance to carry you through.
2. When you start going wide in a turn, push on the inside handlebar to tighten the turn. Having this head knowledge has saved me from crashing numerous times.

SEVENTEEN

Testing Countersteering

Devising a system to convince myself.
— David Mixson

When I started riding, I had a hard time believing the physics of countersteering. It didn't make sense to me. How could I be steering my motorcycle by turning the handlebar in the opposite direction?

To convince myself, I devised a test.

I selected my Honda VFR (the only bike I owned at the time) as my test vehicle and a road south of town (with little traffic and a nice sweeping curve) as my test track.

Early one morning, I headed there by myself and initiated the test.

As I approached the curve, I leaned forward onto my tank bag to the point my body felt rigidly attached to the motorcycle.

The VFR had a forward riding position, which made this easy.

Absolutely Amazing

As I entered the left-handed curve, I pushed on the left handlebar to make the motorcycle lean (turn) to the left.

While I was in the curve, I made small inputs to the handlebar to adjust the turn radius—pushing on the left handlebar to make the bike lean harder, pushing on the right handlebar to make the bike lean less.

After several test runs, something amazing happened—it clicked!

Somehow, taking out all the external factors by leaning onto my tank bag multiplied the sensation, and my brain felt countersteering.

Nonsense to the naysayers who say countersteering doesn't exist. Connect with your motorcycle by leaning over your tank bag and feel what makes your motorcycle turn. COUNTERSTEERING.

WARNING: This test isn't for everyone. It can feel a little unnerving at first. If you start to feel odd, immediately sit up and ride in a normal riding position.

Key Points

1. Countersteering works.
2. Connect with your motorcycle and feel countersteering.

EIGHTEEN

Toys Without Countersteering

Countersteering only works on two-wheeled things that lean to turn.

That means countersteering does NOT work on mechanical stuff such as four-wheelers, Can-AM Spyders, and motorcycle trikes.

Two Examples

On a motorcycle (which uses countersteering), you push left to go left

—or turn the handlebar in the *opposite* direction you want to go.

See Figure 18-1 (below).

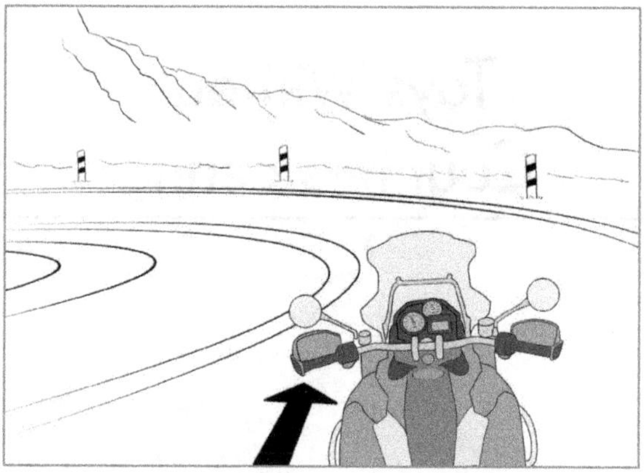

Figure 18-1 Countersteering on Motorcycle (Push on Left Handlebar to Turn Left)

On a Can-AM Spyder (which doesn't use countersteering), you push right to go left—or turn the handlebar in the *same* direction you want to go.

See Figure 18-2 (below).

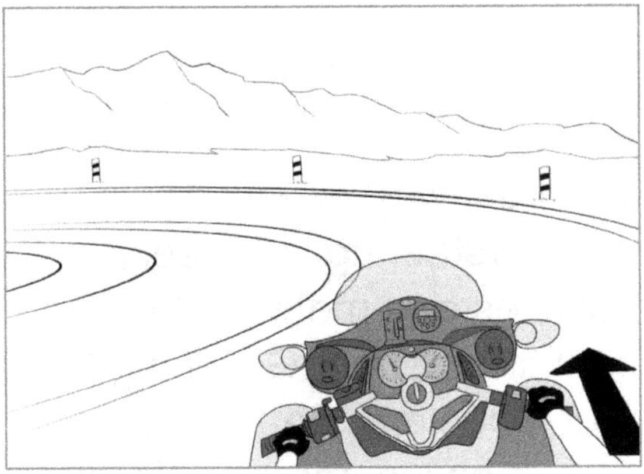

Figure 18-2 Steering on Can-AM Spyder (Push on Right Handlebar to Turn Left)

If you want to feel countersteering, ride something that doesn't use countersteering soon after you've ridden your motorcycle.

You'll notice the difference immediately.

Wasn't that amazing?

The last time I rode my friend's Sea-Doo at his lake house (tough life, right?), it felt awkward. But in a matter of seconds, my brain made the adjustment.

Key Points

1. The best way to believe countersteering is to feel it.
2. Bicycles and motorcycles use countersteering. Goldwing trikes, four-wheelers, Sea-Doos, snowmobiles, motorcycles with sidecars, tractors, trucks, riding lawn mowers, golf carts, and automobiles don't use countersteering.

NINETEEN

Countersteering Wrap-Up

Countersteering is real. Countersteering is how you control your bike.

Countersteering is how you avoid crashing.

Learn how countersteering works (head knowledge), then practice using it until it becomes a part of your muscle memory. Only then can you use it in a pinch to save your life.

If you remember nothing else from this book, remember this:

When you start going wide in a curve:

(1) look where you want to go deep in the curve,

(2) push on the inside handlebar to tighten your turn, and

(3) trust your tires.

THIS DOESN'T HAVE TO FEEL NATURAL ... JUST DO IT. CONGRATULATIONS. YOU JUST PREVENTED A CRASH.

Have you heard about the 'Motorcycle Smarts' Quick Tips Newsletter? I share riding tips (some of which didn't make it into my books) and keep you informed about what's next.

Sign up at the link below.

Unsubscribe at any time.

motorcyclesmarts.com/tips

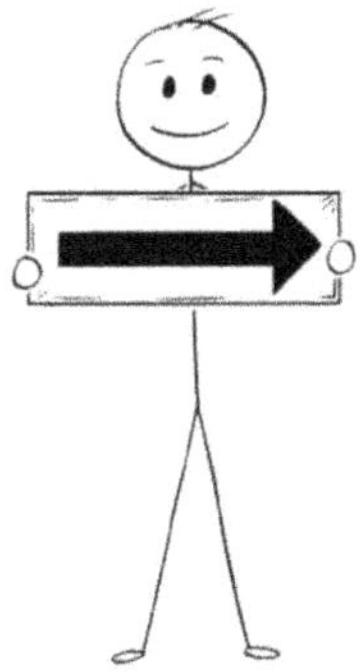

"Motorcycle Smarts" Quick Tips Newsletter

Free weekly riding tips you can consume in less than 3 minutes—delivered to your inbox for you to use and share with others.

motorcyclesmarts.com/tips

You're not doing everything you can to keep from crashing until you're signed up.

Avoid Lowside and Highside Crashes...

and

Outlive Your Riding Buddies

Part Four: Lowside and Highside Crashes

What are they, what causes them, and how you can avoid them?

This might be one of the most in-depth discussions you'll find on the subject of lowside and highside crashes—probably because it's easier to write about how to get the most out of your first motorcycle rally. The information in this section is important because I believe that most lowside and highside crashes are avoidable. I'll explain how.

> NOTE: If you become frustrated with the physics in this section, skip ahead to chapters 28 and 29. There, I'll explain how you can prevent most lowside and highside crashes.

TWENTY

Riding Off My Google Map

Fall is my favorite season of the year and my favorite time to ride.

Every year I forget how Autumn Blaze red maples glow red when the sun hits them just right, how sugar maples burst yellow-orange painting the ground with their leaves—and how the temperature can fluctuate ten degrees in the length of a football field.

I hope heaven is this good.

With a hard rain predicted for Friday, fall color at its peak, and no meetings planned at work, I penciled-in Thursday as *David's Day.* I checked and cross-checked with my wife to make sure she was point for family duties.

My goals for the day were simple: to leave early, enjoy breakfast with a friend, and explore the spectacular fall colors on two-wheels.

I didn't have detailed plans, and that's the way I wanted it.

Before leaving my house, I printed a simple Google map for my tank bag that covered a 30-mile radius. Only a couple of major roads bore numbers on my map, including I-65 that runs north and south.

Mike and I took the long way to breakfast.

We must have passed by two dozen restaurants as we headed south on Highway 431 to Guntersville, Alabama. But that didn't matter.

After a long breakfast, Mike headed to work (something about a meeting to discuss turning astronaut urine into drinking water on the International Space Station), and I headed out solo.

I didn't think much about where I was going. A little south and west seemed good enough. Thirty minutes later, I was outside the parameters of my printed Google map.

Using the inclination of the sun as my guide, I continued. When state roads turned to county, the fun really began. A sign pointed right to Clarkson Covered Bridge. I turned in.

What would normally have been a nice backdrop was no less than spectacular on this beautiful fall day. The deep blue sky and vibrant fall colors were spectacular. After a quick stop, I continued on my adventure through the rural side of Alabama, enjoying every fallen leaf and autumn fragrance. The Elaeagnus shrubs smelled spectacular.

At every intersection, I made a real-time decision to go straight, left, or right. It's hard to describe the joy that overcame me.

I was in the middle of Mother Nature without a map or a clue where I was—and it felt wonderful. I could have stopped for directions (or looked at my GPS), but I didn't want to.

I headed north, then west, then south around Smith Lake.

As I continued, the winding roads became straighter and wider, signaling I was getting close to a city. About that time, a dark green sign with white lettering read "Jasper City Limits."

Alas, I knew where I was, even though I had never been there.

Since it was time to head back to my real life, I started looking for a meaningful road that led east. Highway 69 seemed good enough, so I turned left (heading east and a little north) and clicked up my speed.

Thirty minutes past, I found I-65 and turned left toward home.

I pulled into my garage about an hour later, just in time for my son's Lego Robotics team meeting at my house.

My body felt fatigued. My soul felt rejuvenated.

I got lost today and enjoyed every minute of it.

The Clarkson Covered Bridge is located just off Highway 278 in Cullman County, nine miles west of I-65. The 270-foot bridge (initially built in 1904 for $1500) is one of 14 covered bridges still standing in Alabama.

TWENTY-ONE

Lowside and Highside Crashes

Now that we've mastered countersteering, let's talk about crashing.

In the next several chapters, I'm going to explain lowside and highside crashes, what causes them, and how you can avoid them.

The illustrations are from real crashes captured on video.

Most riders have probably heard of lowside and highside crashes. But I'm going to dial it up a notch and explain how you can virtually eliminate them. Talk about reducing your chances of crashing!

The concepts of lowside and highside crashes aren't that difficult to understand, as long as you don't get bogged down with the physics of how these crashes happen.

However, since there are so many possible scenarios for what triggers these crashes, this section might be the most difficult one to power through in the entire book.

Power through with me.

It's also one of the most important.

Quickie Definitions

Before we get started, here's an introductory definition for each.

In a nutshell, a *lowside* crash is when your motorcycle slides on its side, and you slide on the ground behind it. A *highside* crash is when your bike tosses you up and over the handlebars.

I'll explain both in more detail later in this section.

Just in case I lose you in the details, I want to tell you up-front the most important thing you need to know.

On a motorcycle, BAD THINGS HAPPEN when you lock up (skid) your tires—especially your REAR tire. I feel better knowing I got that point out. It's so important that I'll say it again.

LOCKING UP YOUR REAR TIRE IS BAD.

The topic of lowside and highside crashes is well understood by rider coaches and authors of motorcycle skills books. Yet, most riders don't understand what triggers them.[1] If this is true, our current motorcycle training programs need to be modified.

Here's one man's attempt to thoroughly explain lowside and highside crashes in simple-to-understand language. If you understand and implement the recommendations in this section, you *will* slash your chances of crashing.

TWENTY-TWO

Lowside Crashes

A lowside crash is easier to understand than a highside crash, so let's tackle that one first.

What Is a Lowside?

A lowside crash is when your motorcycle loses stability control, falls on its side sliding, and dumps you (the rider) on the ground behind it. Some refer to a lowside as a "slide-out" because that's sort of what happens—your rear end slides out.

Figure 22-1 (below) shows a rider who has just lowsided.

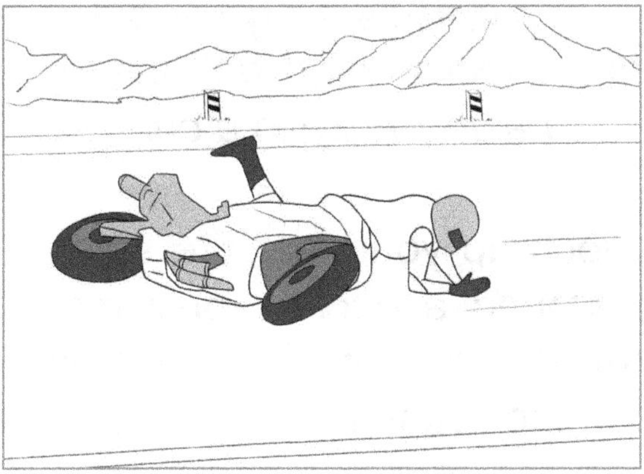

Figure 22-1 Lowside Crash (Motorcycle Slides Out and Dumps Rider)

A lowside occurs when your rear tire (more likely) or front tire (less likely) loses traction with the asphalt. This can happen when you lock up (skid) a tire using your brakes or accelerate too hard in a curve.

NOTE: A skidding tire (which has kinetic friction) has less grip than a rolling tire (which has static friction).

What Triggers Most Lowsides?

Lowside Trigger #1

Rear tire locks up (skids) due to over-braking while in a curve.

If you lock up your rear tire when you're going around a curve, you'll most likely lowside. When your bike is leaning over, it needs the rotational control and friction between the rear tire and the pavement to keep the bike upright.

See Figure 22-2 (below).

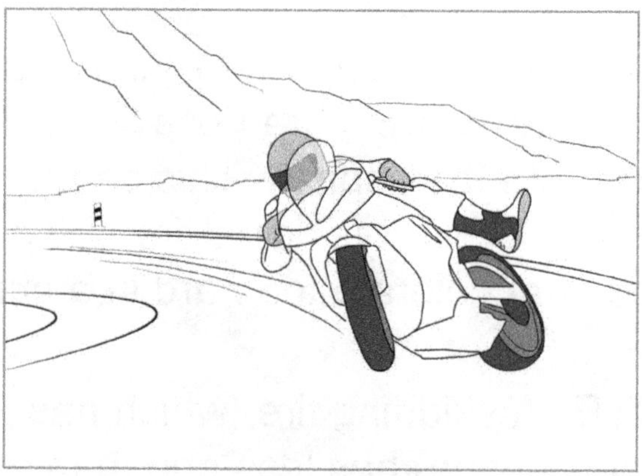

Figure 22-2 Beginning of a Lowside (Rear Tire Locks Up Due to Over-Braking in a Curve)

Once you lose static friction (by locking the rear tire), the back tire will slide out, and the bike will fall on its side —dumping you on the ground behind it.

Lowside Trigger #2

Rear tire locks up (skids) due to over-braking while going straight.

If you lock up your rear tire when you're going in a straight line, you may or may not lowside. It depends on whether the skidding back tire slides around to the side. If the back tire slides around, you'll most likely lowside. If the skidding back tire stays in line with the front tire, you won't lowside.

If you lock up the rear tire when your front brake is applied (likely the case during an emergency stop), or when you're on a road that isn't perfectly flat, the skidding back tire will tend to come around to the side, and you'll most likely lowside.

Lowside Trigger #3

Rear tire spins due to over-accelerating while in a curve.

If you spin your rear tire when you're accelerating hard in a curve (bike is leaned over), you'll most likely lowside because a slipping tire has less friction than a tire in rotational contact with the pavement. Once the rear tire starts slipping, the back end will slide out, and you'll lowside.

Lowside Trigger #4

Front tire locks up (skids) due to over-braking while in a curve.

If you lock up your front tire when you're going around a curve, you'll most likely lowside. When your bike is leaning over, it needs the rotational control and friction between the front tire and the pavement to keep the bike upright.

See Figures 22-3 through 22-5 (below).

NOTE: In the particular example below, the rider wasn't going very fast since neither the rider nor bike slid very far. This isn't always the case. I'll break down a more typical lowside crash in the next chapter.

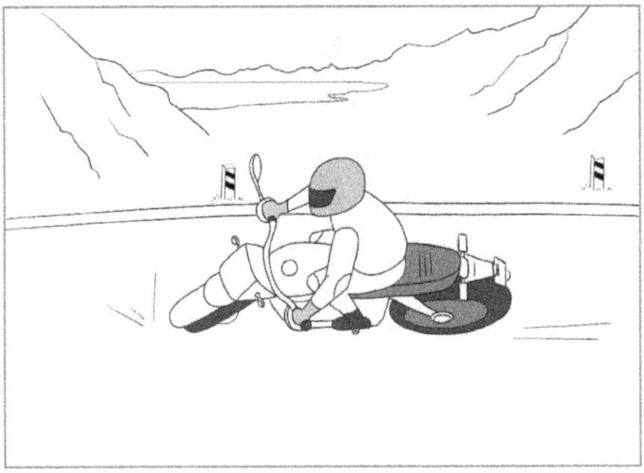

Figure 22-3 Beginning of a Low-Speed Lowside (Front Tire Locks Up Due to Over-Braking in a Curve)

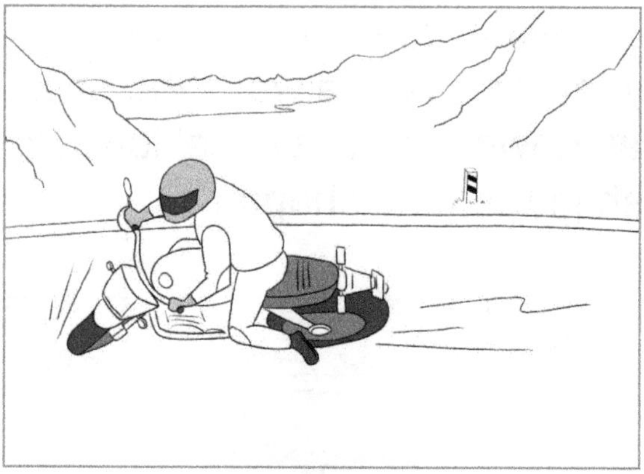

Figure 22-4 Middle of a Low-Speed Lowside (Front Tire Locks Up Due to Over-Braking In a Curve)

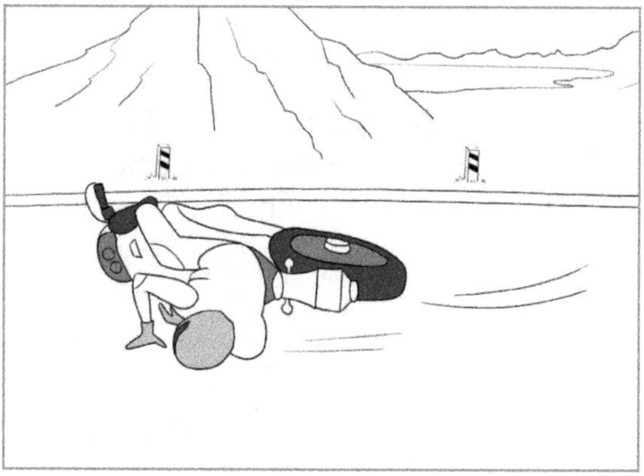

Figure 22-5 End of a Low-Speed Lowside (Front Tire Locks Up Due to Over-Braking in a Curve)

QUICK TIP: It's worth noting that locking up (skidding) your front tire when you're going in a relatively straight line (bike is upright) will NOT cause you to lowside. Tests have shown that a skidding front tire will continue in a straight line as long as the bike is in an upright position.[1] One motorcycle myth debunked.

Locking up (skidding) your *front* tire requires a lot of lever force because weight is transferred to the front tire when you decelerate.

Locking up (skidding) your *rear* tire requires less lever force, especially if you're applying heavy front brake pressure at the same time.

THIS IS WHY LOCKING UP YOUR REAR TIRE IS THE MOST LIKELY TRIGGER FOR A LOWSIDE CRASH.

I've never lowsided, but I've spoken to several riders who have. They all said it happened really fast. In the blink of an eye, they went from *(everything is fine)* to *(my bike is sliding, and I'm sliding behind it)*.

If you think a lowside crash sounds painful, wait until I describe what happens in a highside crash.

> UPDATE: I lowsided on a Backcountry Discovery Route in the George Washington National Forest in Virginia a few years later. The dirt road was a muddy mess. Unfortunately, my bike slid down a 10-foot embankment. My first words after the crash were, "We'll never get it out of there." Two hours later, my riding buddy and I manhandled it up the embankment—only because we didn't have another option. Right as we did, a group came along, and two of the riders lowsided in the exact same spot. I wasn't hurt. *Yes, it happened incredibly fast.*

Key Points

1. A lowside is the same thing as a slide-out.
2. Know what causes a lowside: (1) locking up your rear tire by over-braking (most likely), (2) locking up your front tire while bike is leaned over (less likely), or (3) spinning your rear tire by over-accelerating in a curve (less likely).

TWENTY-THREE

Analysis of a Lowside

Here's a frame-by-frame analysis of a real lowside crash where a rider locked up his rear tire (or over-accelerated) in a curve.

These illustrations are from a *real* crash captured on video.

In Figure 23-1 (below) both tires are in rotational contact with the ground. Everything is working as it should.

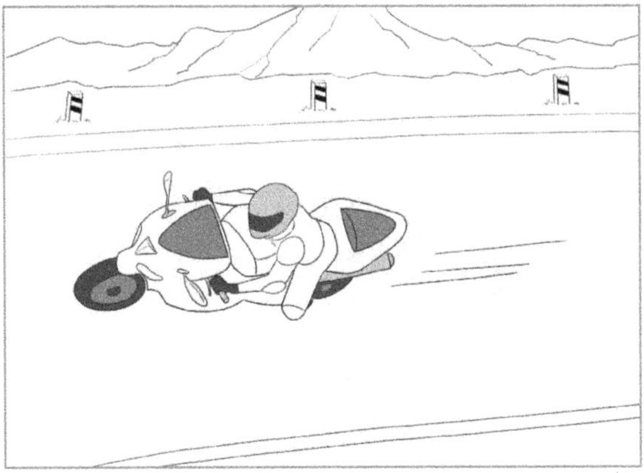

Figure 23-1 Lowside Frame #1
(Riding Around Curve Just Fine)

In Figure 23-2 (below) the rider locks up his rear tire (or over-accelerates and spins rear tire) while he's in the curve.

His rear tire loses rotational contact with the pavement.

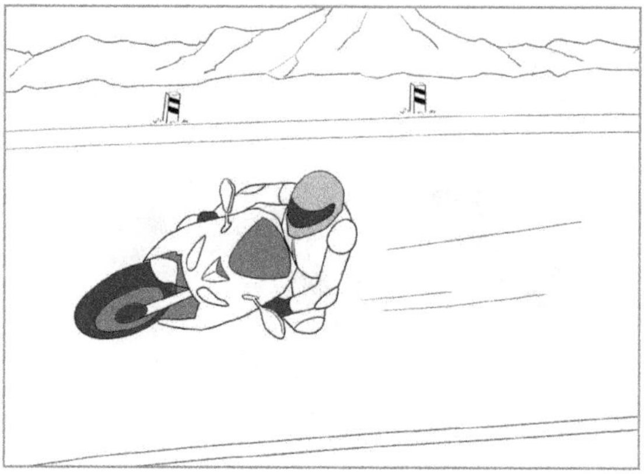

Figure 23-2 Lowside Frame #2
(Rear Tire Loses Traction)

In Figure 23-3 (below) the rear tire starts sliding around. The rider panics and puts his hand down. That won't keep him from crashing.

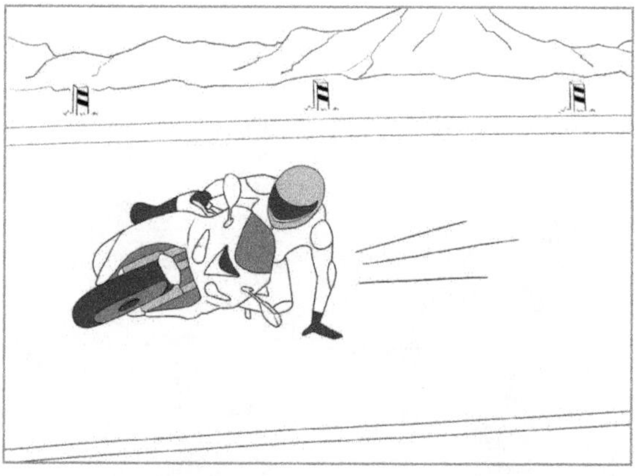

Figure 23-3 Lowside Frame #3
(Rear Tire Slides Around)

In Figure 23-4 (below) the motorcycle slides and dumps rider.

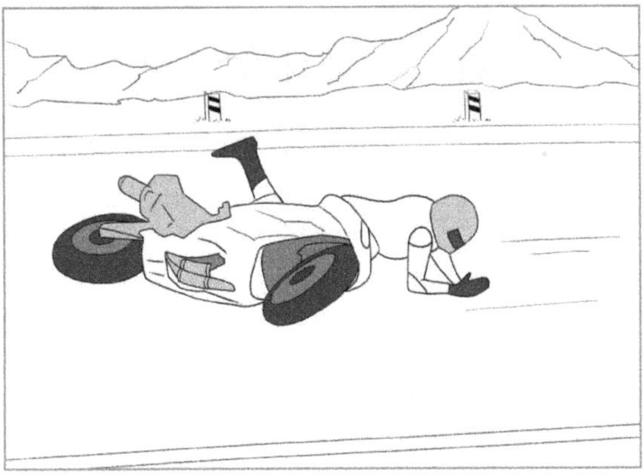

Figure 23-4 Lowside Frame #4 (Bike on Side and Rider Dumped)

In Figure 23-5 (below) the rider and motorcycle continue sliding. How far each slides depends on how fast the rider was going when he lowsided, and how easily the bike and rider slide on the ground.

Let's hope the motorcycle slides more easily (often the case) so the rider won't slide into the back of his sliding bike.

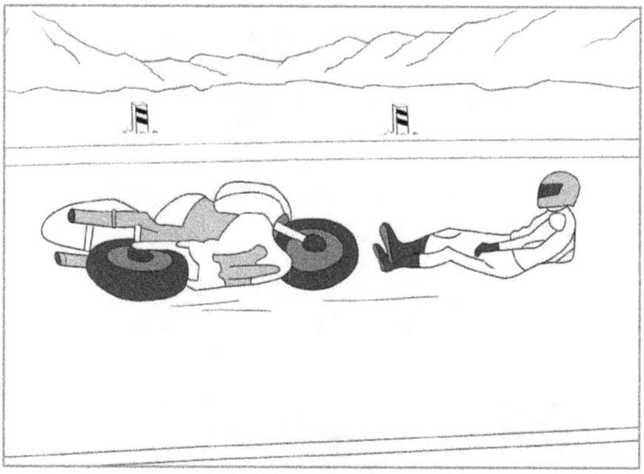

Figure 23-5 Lowside Frame #5 (Bike and Rider Slide)

In Figure 23-6 (below) the motorcycle and rider come to a stop. In this example, the rider stopped faster than his motorcycle. Good news.

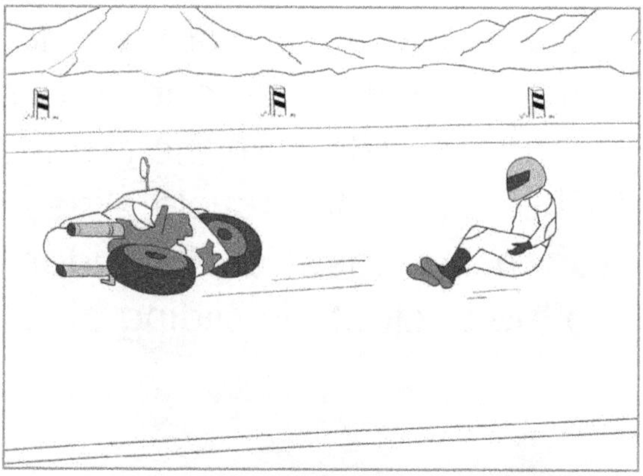

Figure 23-6 Lowside Frame #6 (Bike and Rider Stop)

THERE YOU HAVE IT ... A FRAME-BY-FRAME ANALYSIS OF AN ACTUAL LOWSIDE CRASH.

Key Points

1. Most lowsides end with the rider sliding behind his bike.
2. Jeans won't help much if you lowside, but abrasion-resist riding gear (jacket, pants, and gloves) could.
3. There's good news ahead. Most lowside and highside crashes can be prevented with electronics. Keep reading.

TWENTY-FOUR

Highside Crashes

The thought of highsiding makes me want to sell my motorcycle.
— David Mixson

Now that we understand lowside crashes and what causes them, let's look at highside crashes. I've spent hours going through slow-motion videos trying to understand the physics of a highside.

And this is what I've discovered.

I have to warn you. What you're about to learn is both *fascinating* and *terrifying*. The physics of a highside is fascinating!

The thought of doing a highside is terrifying!

What Is a Highside?

A highside crash is when your motorcycle loses stability control and catapults you over the handlebars. You eventually hit the ground, often headfirst, and your bike tumbles toward you.

Figure 24-1 (below) shows a rider in the middle of a highside.

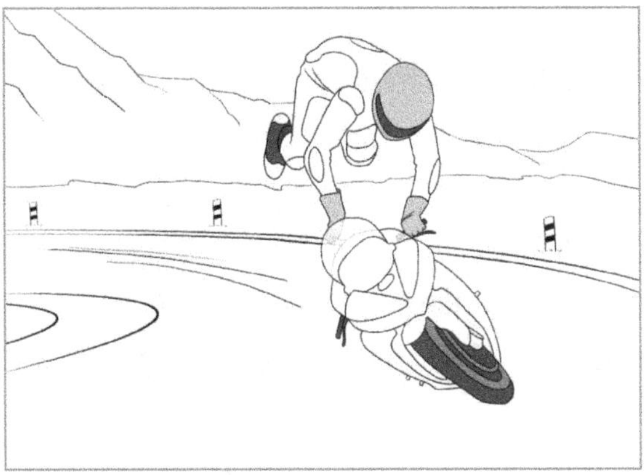

Figure 24-1 Highside Crash
(Motorcycle Catapults Rider)

Yeah, I know. Freaking scary, right?

A highside occurs when a skidding rear tire, which has slid out of alignment with the front tire, is released and allowed to rotate again.

Why It Happens

When the rear brake is released, the skidding rear tire (which has now slid out of alignment with the front) starts rotating again and immediately tracks inline behind the front tire. When this happens, the bike instantly sits up to a vertical position.

Since the motorcycle was leaned over (squatted) because the rear tire was sliding, the motion of the motorcycle snapping to a vertical position is like releasing a coiled-up spring.

This combination launches the rider into the air.

NOTE: I know this is a hard concept to understand. It's also a hard one to explain. I must be on my hundredth edit of this section. Stay with me. I have real examples (below and in the next chapter) that I think will help.

In Figure 24-2 (below) the skidding rear tire has moved out of alignment with the front. If the rider releases the rear brake and allows the tire to rotate again, he will most likely highside.

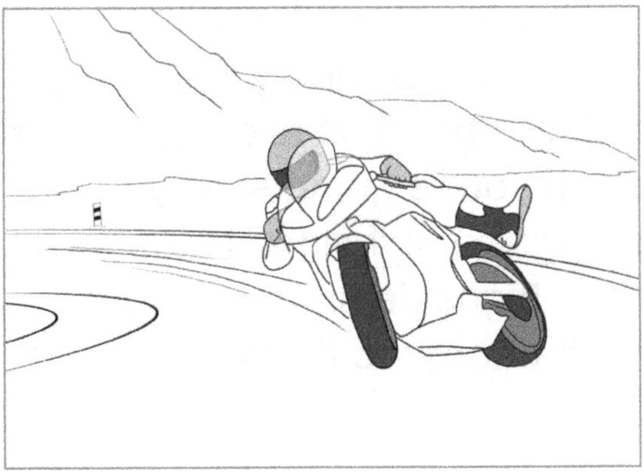

Figure 24-2 Rear Tire Slides Out

What Triggers Most Highsides?

Highside Trigger #1

Locking up rear tire (and then releasing it) while in a curve.

If you lock up (skid) your rear tire (by over-braking) while going around a curve, then release the rear brake and allow the tire to rotate again, you'll most likely highside.

> QUICK TIP: The faster you're going when you lock up your rear tire (and the farther out the skidding rear tire gets while it's locked up), the more abruptly the rear end will snap up once the rear tire is allowed to rotate again. If you're going slowly when you trigger a highside, it's unlikely that the highside snap will have enough energy to throw you off your bike.

Highside Trigger #2

Spinning rear tire (and then backing off throttle) while in a curve.

If you spin your rear tire (by over-accelerating) when going around a curve, then back off the throttle and allow the tire to regain traction, you'll most likely highside.

Highside Trigger #3

Locking up rear tire (and then releasing it) while on a straight road.

Unfortunately, you don't have to be in a curve to highside.

Let's assume you're making an emergency stop and applying both front and rear brakes. Since you're stopping so quickly, weight is transferred to the front of the bike.

Good, because it gives your front tire more stopping power.

Not so good, because it takes load off your rear tire (which makes it easier to lock up).

If you lock up your rear tire while you are braking hard with your front brake, the skidding back tire can skid around to the side because the front tire is braking hard and the skidding rear tire lost directional control and static friction.

Now you're in trouble. If you then release the rear brake and allow the tire to rotate again, you'll most likely highside.

Here's the dilemma. Once your back tire starts skidding (by over-braking), or spinning (by over-accelerating), one of two things is likely to happen: You'll either LOWSIDE or HIGHSIDE.

I'm getting depressed thinking about my options.

While I have your attention, let me say it (again) because it's one of the most important points in this entire book.

LOCKING UP YOUR REAR TIRE IS BAD BECAUSE IT TRIGGERS MOST LOWSIDE AND HIGHSIDE CRASHES.

Key Points

1. A highside almost always starts the same way as a lowside.

2. I know this is a hard concept to understand. That's why I'm going to take two real examples and break them down (frame-by-frame) in the next chapter.

TWENTY-FIVE

Analysis of a Highside

Here's a frame-by-frame analysis of two real highside crashes where the rider locked up his rear tire (or over-accelerated) in a curve and then allowed the tire to start rolling normally again (by releasing the brake or backing off the throttle). Remember, these are freeze-frame illustrations of *real* crashes that were captured on video.

Highside Crash Example #1

In Figure 25-1 (below) both tires are in strong rotational contact with the ground. Everything is good.

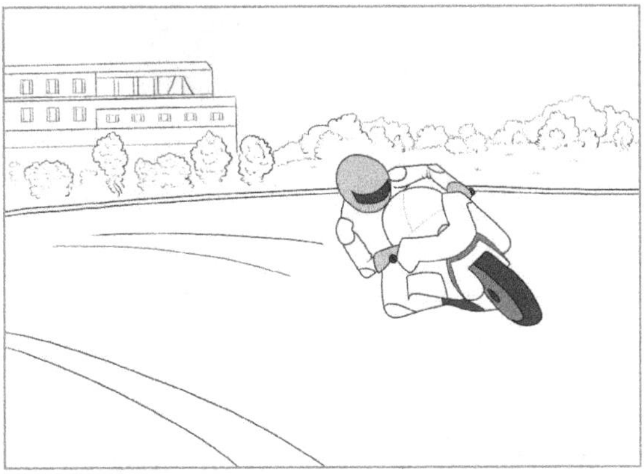

Figure 25-1 Highside Frame #1
(Riding Around Curve Just Fine)

In Figure 25-2 (below) the back end starts to slide out in the curve because the rear tire has lost rotational contact with the asphalt. This is because the rear tire is either locked up (from over-braking), or spinning (from over-accelerating).

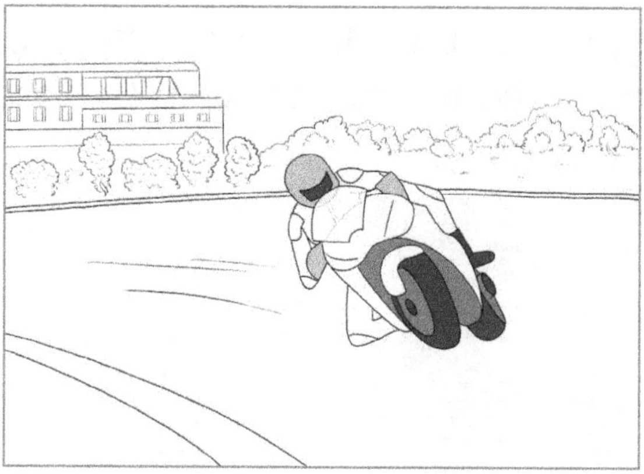

Figure 25-2 Highside Frame #2
(Rear Tire Slides Around)

In Figure 25-3 (below) it looks like the rider has released the rear brake (or let off the throttle) and allowed the rear tire to rotate again. The rear tire is trying to get back in alignment with the front tire.

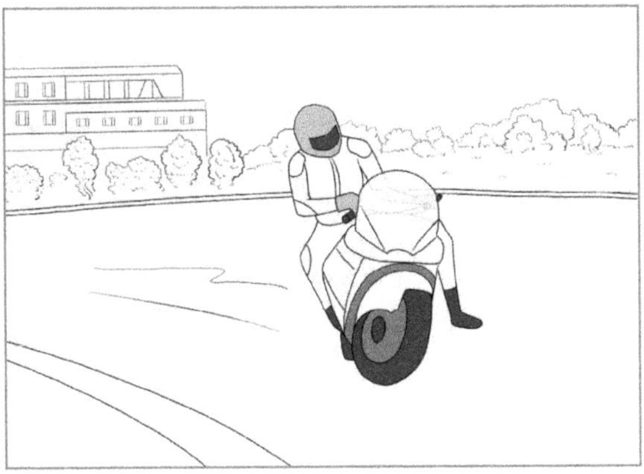

Figure 25-3 Highside Frame #3
(Rear Tire Regains Traction)

In Figure 25-4 (below) the rear tire is rotating again, and the bike has snapped up into a vertical position. This motion catapults the rider up into the air off his motorcycle.

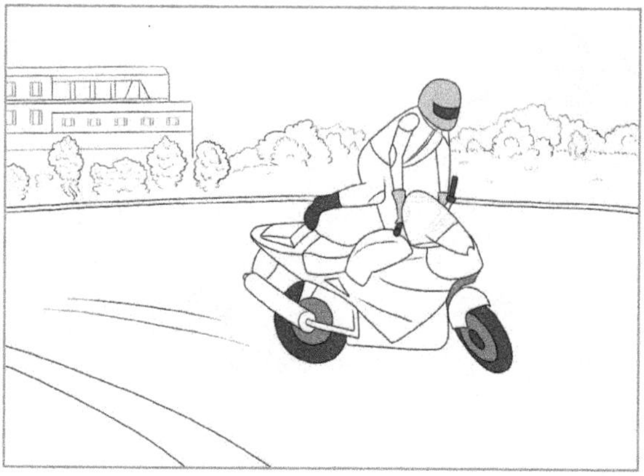

Figure 25-4 Highside Frame #4
(Bike Launches Rider)

In Figure 25-5 (below) the fun doesn't stop. The rider flies over the handlebars, and his motorcycle becomes unstable.

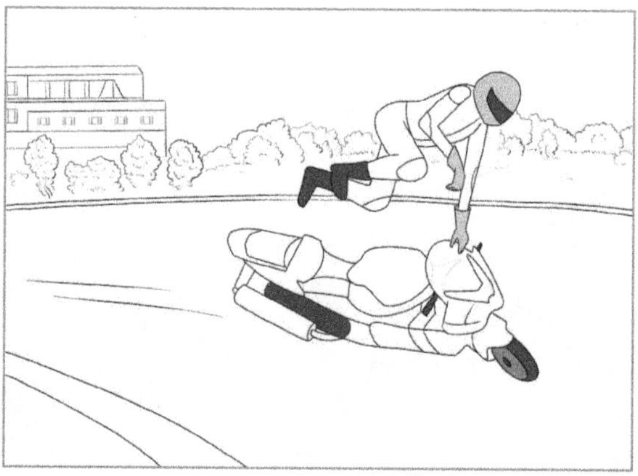

Figure 25-5 Highside Frame #5
(Bike Becomes Unstable)

In Figure 25-6 (below) the rider heads toward the asphalt, and his motorcycle starts tumbling.

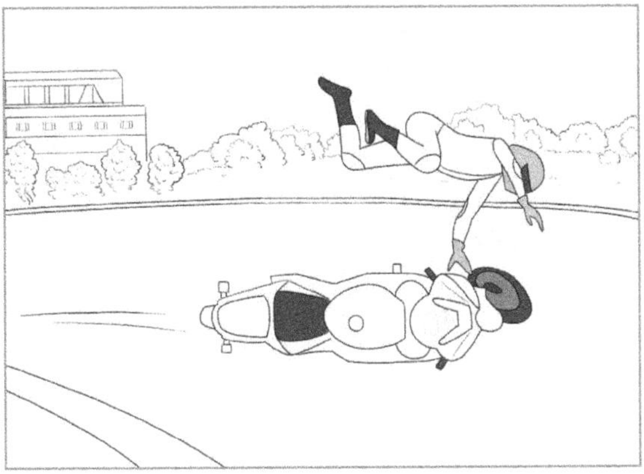

Figure 25-6 Highside Frame #6
(Rider Prays)

In Figure 25-7 (below) the rider reaches the ground, and his bike tumbles toward him.

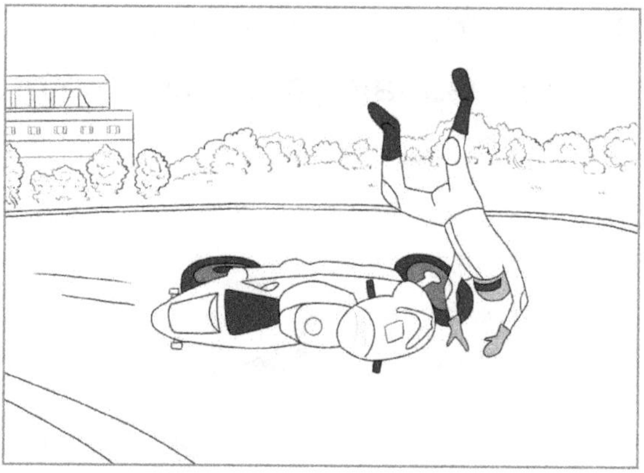

Figure 25-7 Highside Frame #7
(Rider Lands)

Doing a highside doesn't look very fun, but studying the physics sure is. Let's take a look at another one!

Highside Crash Example #2

This highside is a little different but just as real. In Figure 25-8 (below) both tires are in solid rotational contact with the ground.

Everything is good.

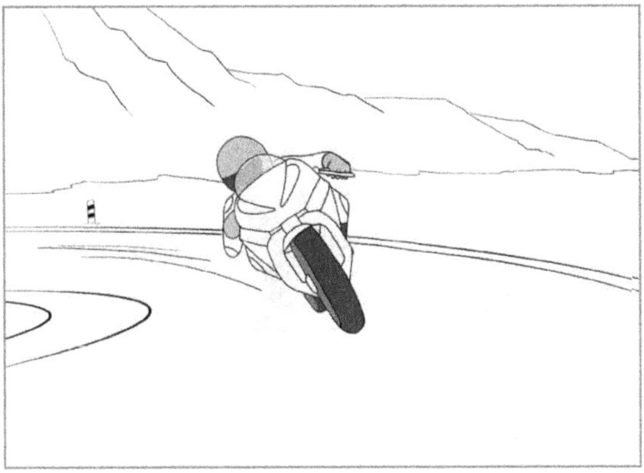

Figure 25-8 Highside Frame #1
(Riding Around Curve Just Fine)

In Figure 25-9 (below) the back end starts to slide out in the curve because the rear tire has lost rotational contact with the asphalt. This is because the rear tire is either locked up (from over-braking), or spinning (from over-accelerating).

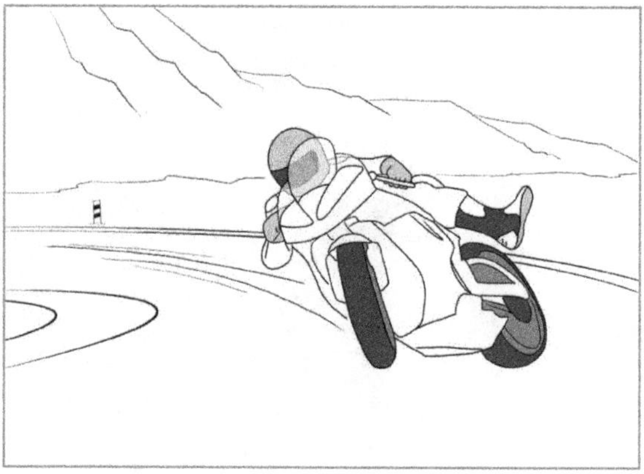

Figure 25-9 Highside Frame #2
(Rear Tire Slides Around)

In Figure 25-10 (below) the rear tire is rotating again, and the bike has snapped up into a vertical position.

This motion catapults the rider into the air.

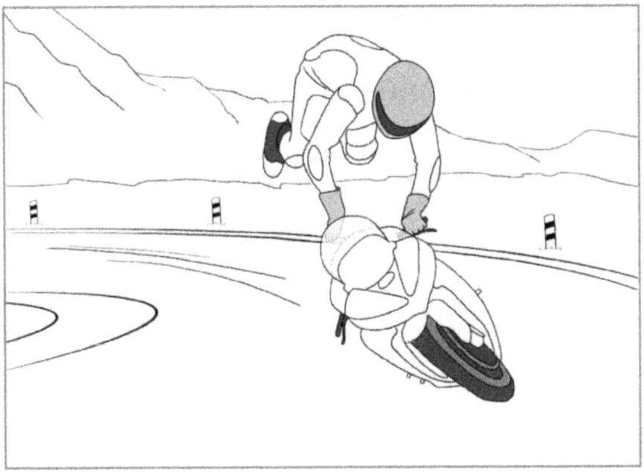

Figure 25-10 Highside Frame #3
(Bike Launches Rider)

In Figure 25-11 (below) the fun continues. The rider flies over the handlebars, and his bike keeps going.

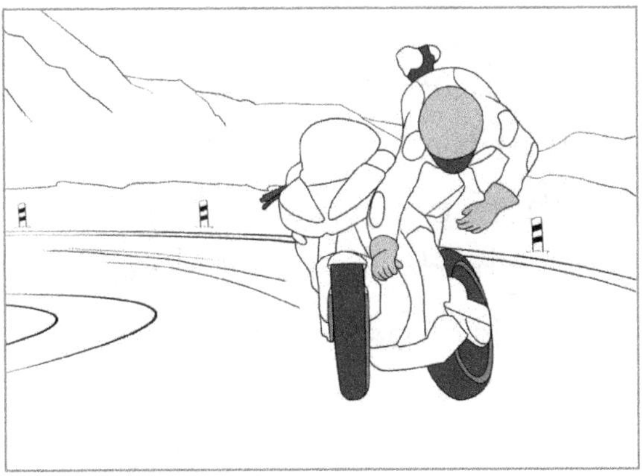

Figure 25-11 Highside Frame #4
(Bike Remains Stable)

In Figure 25-12 (below) the rider lands, and his bike heads away from him (fortunately).

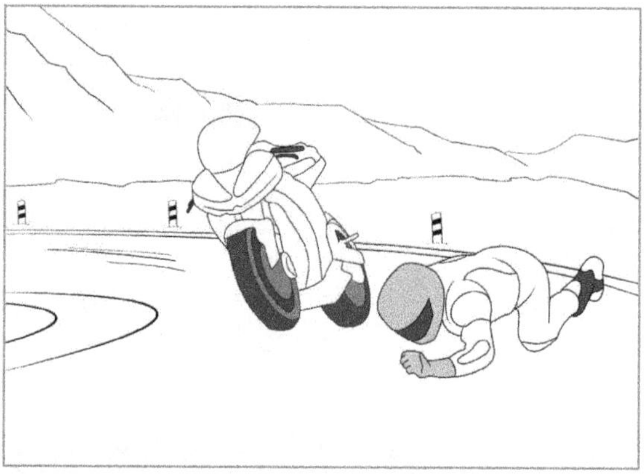

Figure 25-12 Highside Frame #5
(Rider Lands)

There you have it ... a frame-by-frame analysis of two real highside crashes. I suppose there are worse things in life than doing a highside, but exactly what those might be escapes me.

Key Points

1. Most highsides end with the rider being thrown into the air off his motorcycle.
2. Highside crashes look incredibly uncomfortable. Thank goodness, I can base that only on speculation.
3. There's good news ahead. Most lowside and highside crashes can be prevented with electronics. Keep reading.

TWENTY-SIX

Lowside and Highside Examples

Now that we understand what lowside and highside crashes are, let's look at more examples. The scenarios below are my attempt to think through what might happen in a lowside or highside crash.

I'm confident not everyone will agree with my assessments. They're not meant to be absolutes of what will happen. Instead, they're meant to help us understand what causes most lowsides and highsides.

Once we understand the causes, we can better avoid them.

Scenario #1

In this example, let's assume a rider is on a straight, flat road and is NOT using his front brake. The rider could probably lock up his rear tire and skid to a stop without lowsiding. This is because the back end has no force (front-tire braking or uneven road) to make it slide to the side of the bike when it's skidding.

The rider could most likely release his skidding rear tire without highsiding. Why? Because as long as he can keep the skidding rear tire in line (behind) the front tire, nothing significant will happen when the rear tire is allowed to rotate again.

> NOTE: While it might sound like I'm suggesting that using *only* your rear brake might be a good thing, *I'm not.* Without going into all the details here (more on braking comes in later chapters), I'll quickly make the point that stopping power on your rear tire is only a fraction of your front, making it incredibly easy to lock up your rear

tire under heavy braking (the exact thing we're trying to avoid because it initiates most lowside and highside crashes).

Scenario #2

In this example, let's assume a rider is on a perfectly flat, straight road and is applying heavy braking (both front and rear) to avoid an object. If the rider locks up his rear tire, the back end will most likely slide around to the side of the motorcycle because the front tire is under heavy braking.

At this point, if the rider keeps the rear tire locked up, he will most likely lowside. If he releases the rear brake after the rear tire starts skidding, he will most likely highside.

Scenario #3

In this example, let's assume a rider is on a straight road that is slanted to allow water to runoff, and that he is NOT using his front brake. If the rider locks up his rear tire, the back end of the motorcycle might slide around on the downhill side of the road.

If the back tire slides to the side and the rider keeps the rear tire locked up, he will most likely lowside. If he releases the rear brake after the back tire has slid to the side, he will most likely highside.

In this scenario, I can also imagine a situation where the skidding rear tire didn't go around to the side, and instead tracked behind the front tire. If this happens, no lowside or highside.

Scenario #4

In this example, let's assume a rider is in a sharp curve. If he locks up his rear tire, he will most likely lowside immediately because the rear tire will slide out quickly in a curve. If he is quick enough to release the rear brake before he lowsides, he will most likely highside.

> WARNING: It's difficult to recover from a locked-up rear tire when

you're going around a curve because the back end tends to slide out so fast. If you're quick enough to save a lowside, you'll be greeted with an energy-packed highside launch. This is because the motorcycle is leaned over and low to the ground (like a coiled-up spring) when it highside-snaps.

QUICK TIP: It's probably worth noting *again* that your *speed* when you lock up your rear tire determines how likely you are to lowside or highside. Speed translates into energy. If you're only going 20 mph, it's unlikely the energy of the highside-snap will be enough to throw you off your bike. Highsides for MotoGP racers going 200 mph look entirely different. The highside snap is brutal and nearly instant.

Key Points

1. These examples are intended to make you think. It's difficult to know exactly what would happen in each scenario because there are so many external factors.
2. If you lock up your rear tire in a curve, chances are higher that you'll lowside (or highside) than if you lock up your rear tire riding in a straight line on even pavement.

TWENTY-SEVEN

Recovering Options

The prospects aren't very promising.
— DAVID MIXSON

Now that we understand what lowside and highside crashes are (and what causes them), let's take it a step further and answer the question:

What should you do if your rear tire starts to skid?

You have several options.

Option #1

Since a highside is worse than a lowside, some suggest that you keep your rear wheel locked up until you either regain control (less likely) or do a lowside (more likely). While this doesn't sound very appealing to me, I can understand the logic.

I suppose.

Option #2

Some suggest that turning the handlebar in the direction the rear tire is sliding out will increase the chances you might recover.

This might be true, but I've seen numerous videos where the rider did this and still lowsided or highsided.

Option #3

Some suggest that if you release a skidding rear tire immediately after it starts skidding (by releasing the rear brake or getting off the throttle), you might be able to avoid a lowside and highside crash.

> QUICK TIP: The likelihood of this working depends on how fast you're going, whether you're using your front brake at the time, and how far out of alignment your rear tire has gotten during the skid. Remember, as long as your skidding rear tire tracks behind your front tire, it's unlikely that you will lowside or highside.

Option #4

Some suggest that putting your weight on the outside peg (loading it) right when your rear tire locks up might keep you from highsiding.

I contacted a rider that I saw highside crash on YouTube. He told me that he put all his weight on the outside peg right when his rear tire started skidding. He highsided anyway.

NOTE: While the options above might help, I'm just not convinced they'll keep you from crashing if your skidding rear tire has gotten out of alignment with your front tire.

Here's the dilemma that plagues me at night.

Once you've locked up your rear tire (the trigger in most lowside and highside crashes), you must decide (quickly) what to do next.

If you immediately release the rear brake, you will either recover or highside—and probably hit the object you're braking for.

If you hold the rear brake, you will either recover or lowside.

What should you do? I can't answer that question for you. Mostly because I can't answer it for MYSELF.

Key Points

1. If you lock up your rear tire, what are you going to do?
2. There's good news ahead. Most lowside and highside crashes can be prevented with electronics. Keep reading.

TWENTY-EIGHT

Preventing Lowside and Highside Crashes

In this section, we've established two things: (1) a skidding rear tire is the trigger that causes most lowside and highside crashes, and (2) once your rear tire starts to skid, you don't have any plausible options to keep from crashing.

Now that we understand this (head knowledge), we need a way to keep from skidding (over-braking and over-accelerating) our rear tire.

Well, there's the obvious: maintain your tires, ride with margin, slow down before the turn so you won't have to brake in the turn, and be easy on the throttle while you're in a turn.

But even better, there's something else you can do that will significantly reduce the chances of a lowside or highside crash.

RIDE A MOTORCYCLE EQUIPPED WITH AN ANTI-LOCK BRAKING SYSTEM (ABS).

ABS is an electronic system that prevents your tires from locking up. When the ABS detects that a tire is about to lock up, it automatically reduces brake pressure to that tire.

ABS has been standard on cars for years.

While ABS virtually eliminates most lowside and highside crashes due to over-braking, it doesn't keep you from spinning (over-accelerating) your rear tire in a curve.

But the story doesn't end here.

There's another piece of electronics, called *Traction Control*, that keeps your rear tire from spinning-out while accelerating.

Isn't this great news!

Traction Control uses the ABS sensors on both tires to detect when the rear tire starts to rotate faster than the front tire. When this state is detected, the system cuts power to the engine to prevent the rear wheel from spinning out. I'll explain Traction Control in a later chapter.

Here's the awesome truth: ABS and Traction Control can prevent certain types of crashes—and almost certainly save lives!

If this is true, why doesn't every motorcycle have them?

Good question. I'll attempt to answer that a little later.

WARNING: ABS and Traction Control can't overcome physics. If you're going around a curve faster than your tires can handle (or hit a slippery spot), you're going down.

ABS and Traction Control don't give you more friction, but they do significantly reduce your chances of crashing.

Key Points

1. The best way to eliminate most lowside and highside crashes is to ride a bike with ABS and Traction Control.
2. Don't listen to the naysayers who say otherwise.

TWENTY-NINE

Lowside and Highside Wrap-Up

This section was my best attempt to explain what I think every rider should know about lowside and highside crashes.

If you're mentally exhausted, I feel your pain.

The subject of lowside crashes and highside crashes (what are they, what triggers them, and how you can prevent them) is one of the most *glossed over* topics in motorcycling. I spent a great deal of time writing this section because I think the information can make you a safer rider.

I know I can't convince everyone to purchase a motorcycle with ABS and Traction Control, but I wish I could. Two little pieces of electronics could eliminate most lowside and highside crashes.

I'm a believer.

If you're serious about avoiding lowside and highside crashes, ride with margin, maintain your tires, watch your speed when entering a curve, be easy on the throttle, and …

RIDE A MOTORCYCLE EQUIPPED WITH ABS AND TRACTION CONTROL (or ESC).

If you do these things, you *will* reduce your chances of crashing.

And you *might* even outlive your riding buddies.

Crashes Leave Clues

Part Five: Electronics, Braking, and the Hurt Report

Now that we understand lowside crashes and highside crashes—and what causes them—let's move on to something a little easier. While this section isn't as technical, the information is just as important.

In the next several chapters, I'll expand on our earlier discussion of how electronics can help us ride more safely. I'll also discuss proper braking techniques and how we can all reduce our risk of crashing by learning from riders who have already crashed.

Congratulations for sticking with me.

We're on the downhill side of the mountain now.

THIRTY

Mid-Life and Motorbikes

I'm not sure there's any truth to the hypothesis that men buy motorcycles during their mid-life crisis.

Sure, I was 40 when I purchased my first motorcycle, but I don't think I was going through a mid-life crisis. That came later. I was merely at a point in my life where owning a motorcycle made more sense. My kids were older, I wasn't getting any younger, and my bank account said I could pay cash and still keep my life insurance current.

Apparently, I'm not the only one coming to this conclusion.

I get emails often from listeners of the *Motorcycle Mentor Podcast* who have decided to take up riding later in life—some in their 40s, some in their 50s, and some even in their 60s.

It makes sense when you think about it. We all reach a point in life (hopefully) when our kids can take care of themselves, and we are still in good enough mental and physical health to explore.

This season in life begs to be enjoyed.

On second thought, maybe buying a motorcycle during your mid-life crisis is the perfect time.

The excuse certainly helped me convince my wife.

THIRTY-ONE

Arguments Against ABS

If you've listened to the *Motorcycle Mentor Podcast*, you know I like to present both sides of every argument. I've already presented the *advantages* of ABS. In this chapter, I'll present the *disadvantages*.

Nearly all new cars and trucks sold in the United States come with ABS as standard equipment.

The technology is simple, mature, and relatively inexpensive.

So why haven't motorcycle manufacturers embraced ABS like the automotive industry?

Simple economics suggests it's because riders aren't demanding it.

Hopefully, this book will change a few minds.

Before we dive in, let me assure you that none of the arguments I'm about to present sway my strong belief that motorcycles equipped with ABS are significantly safer than motorcycles without.

ABS Disadvantage #1

The argument against ABS I hear most often is this.

"A friend said my first motorcycle shouldn't have ABS because it encourages poor braking habits."

My Thoughts:

ABS allows you to grab (squeeze) more brake than you could with conventional brakes. But just because you have ABS doesn't mean you will be forced to brake incorrectly. ABS doesn't change the way you brake; it just keeps you from locking up your tires.

The most important thing to know about motorcycle braking is that you should *predominantly use your front brake.* A bike without ABS won't teach you this, and it certainly won't slap you on the butt when you use your rear brake too much. The second most important thing to know about proper motorcycle braking is that you should *avoid locking up your rear tire.* ABS keeps you from doing this.

Proper braking techniques are first learned with your head and then developed with practice and repetition until the "correct way" becomes a part of your muscle memory.

This process is the same whether you have ABS or not.

More on correct braking techniques in a later chapter.

ABS Disadvantage #2

The second argument against ABS I hear is this.

"Some riders can stop faster on a motorcycle without ABS than they can on the same motorcycle equipped with ABS."

My Thoughts:

This might be true for top riders. But while we would all like to believe we're in the top rider category, few of us are. I'm certainly not, and I presume you're not either. I'm not particularly motivated that MotoGP champion Valentino Rossi can stop faster *without* ABS.

I'm more moved that you and I can stop more quickly *with* ABS.

Every study I've seen shows that most riders (from beginning to experienced) can stop more quickly in panic situations with ABS than without it. As ABS technology improves, I predict that even MotoGP racers will use it. I promise they understand what's going to happen if their rear tire loses traction at 200 mph.

Hello, highside!

ABS Disadvantage #3

The third argument against ABS I hear is this.

"Motorcycles with ABS don't perform as well in dirt and gravel."

My Thoughts:

There's some truth to this argument, but it's not always the case. Some tests actually show that motorcycles with ABS stop just as well or even better than their non-ABS cousins in off-road situations.[1]

Many adventure motorcycles like the BMW R1200GS Adventure (my current bike), allow the rider to disengage the ABS.

Perfect. Turn ABS "off" when you go off-road—if you want to.

> NOTE: I usually keep my ABS "on" even when I'm riding in off-road conditions. But that discussion is for another book.

The Bottom Line

I don't profess that current ABS technology is perfect. But the advantages—shorter stopping distances, fewer lowside and highside crashes, easier to use in panic stops—far outweigh the disadvantages. So much so that I've made a personal commitment never to own a modern bike that doesn't have ABS.

Just last week I spotted a beautiful used Ducati ST4 for sale. The owner really wanted to sell it and marked it down to a great price.

I wanted it, but it didn't have ABS.

I had a serious conversation with myself and decided not to buy it.

I'll wait for one that has ABS.

Stop for a moment and think about it this way. If a car spinning out of control is coming across your lane in front of you, do you really want to worry about grabbing the *correct* amount of front and rear brake—the amount that stops you in the shortest distance but doesn't lock up your rear tire?

I don't ... and I won't ... because I have ABS.

I can grab both brakes and let ABS do its thing.

My Best Advice ... CHOOSE A MOTORCYCLE WITH ABS.

BMW embraced ABS before most. When I started looking for my first motorcycle, the only used motorcycles with ABS in my price range (motorcycles old enough) were BMWs.

I didn't fully understand the advantages of ABS back then, so I ended up buying a motorcycle with conventional brakes.

BMW continues to lead the way. In 2013 BMW Motorrad was the first manufacturer to equip all new motorcycles with ABS as standard equipment. Way to go BMW.

ABS has been available on most touring and sport-touring bikes for years. Recently, other manufacturers (including Harley Davidson) have started offering models with ABS—sometimes as standard equipment and sometimes as an upgrade.

That's awesome.

I want my Harley friends to have the same advantages that I do.

If you want to significantly reduce your chances of crashing, DITCH the LOUD PIPES and RIDE A HARLEY WITH ABS. Your neighbors might even love you for it.

Key Points

1. Embrace ABS. The advantages outweigh the disadvantages.
2. The worst braking habit is overusing your rear brake.
3. Don't listen to anyone who says ABS is bad. You don't have to argue with them. Just ignore them. Better yet, hand them a copy of this book and smile.

THIRTY-TWO

The Wrong Argument for ABS

Now that we've established that ABS is a beautiful thing, let's take a look at why some riders still don't see its benefits.

ABS proponents argue that ABS shortens their stopping distance, while anti-ABS proponents argue that top riders can stop more quickly with conventional brakes.

In this case, neither side wins because both sides are right.

WE'RE LOSING THE ABS DEBATE BECAUSE WE'RE USING THE WRONG ARGUMENT.

The main reason I like ABS has nothing to do with stopping distances and everything to do with something we discussed earlier—crashing. In my mind, the real benefit of ABS is that it *eliminates most lowside and highside crashes*.

Another benefit I rarely hear mentioned is that riders with ABS feel less stress in panic stops because they don't have to worry about braking correctly. In other words, they can squeeze both brakes firmly without fear of locking up either tire.

This allows riders to focus more on avoiding the obstacle they're braking for in the first place.

According to an NHTSA study:

> *"Anti-lock brake systems not only prevent rider and motorcycle from harm and damage by increasing active safety, but also reduce significantly [the] mental strain while*

riding and braking. In case of a critical riding situation, this higher remaining mental reserve would help the rider to develop and wishfully realize alternative emergency strategies that additionally could help the rider to prevent a crash."[1]

NOW YOU KNOW THE REAL REASON I ONLY OWN MOTORCYCLES WITH ABS

Key Points

1. Want to win the ABS debate? Instead of arguing that ABS will shorten your stopping distance, argue that ABS will eliminate most lowside and highside crashes, and reduce mental strain in emergency situations.

2. Don't be the guy who lets pride stand in your way of getting a bike with ABS. Having ABS doesn't make you a wimp. It signals that you know what you're talking about. It shows that you give a damn about your riding safety.
3. Once you've MASTERED THE ART OF RIDING WELL, the single best thing you can do to reduce your chances of crashing is to ride a motorcycle equipped with ABS.

THIRTY-THREE

Insurance and Mandatory ABS

I'm not the only one who likes motorcycles with ABS.

Insurance companies love them too because riders on motorcycles with ABS file fewer claims than riders on motorcycles without ABS.

That's saying something.

The statistical data is so overwhelming that the Insurance Institute for Highway Safety and the Highway Loss Data Institute have asked the NHTSA to make ABS mandatory on all street motorcycles manufactured in the United States.

> *"The letter addressed to David Strickland, NHTSA Administrator, included a recent IIHS study on the effects of ABS on motorcycle fatal crash rates. The report found that ABS technology reduces the rate of fatal crashes by 31 percent, while collision claim rates were 20 percent lower with ABS-equipped motorcycles."*[1]

Beginning in 2016, the European Parliament approved regulations that made ABS mandatory on all new street motorcycles over 125cc. India, Japan, and Brazil have also approved legislation to make ABS mandatory on certain sizes of motorcycles.

Meanwhile, ABS legislation for motorcycles pops up on the political agenda in the U.S. and Australia from time to time.

Mandatory ABS for motorcycles is coming soon to a country near you. As far as I'm concerned, this is EXCELLENT news.

Key Points

1. Insurance companies have studied the data. Motorcycles with ABS crash less often than motorcycles without ABS.
2. I predict that ABS will someday be required on all street motorcycles sold in the United States. In my lifetime?

THIRTY-FOUR

Traction Control and Stability Control

Now that we understand the importance of ABS on motorcycles, let's talk about other electronics that can reduce your chances of crashing.

Recall that ABS keeps you from skidding your tires when braking (a leading trigger of lowside and highside crashes), but it doesn't keep you from spinning your rear tire when over-accelerating in a curve (also a trigger of lowside and highside crashes).

I have good news. *Traction Control* will.

Traction Control is an electronic system that prevents your rear tire from spinning (losing rotational contact with the asphalt) when accelerating. The system uses the ABS sensors to detect when your rear tire is slipping. When it does, it reduces torque to the rear wheel by cutting engine power.

Traction Control can also help you maintain control in low-speed situations like pulling out from a side street over a high lip of asphalt.

Remember, your rear tire has less friction once it starts spinning and wants to slide around to the side of least resistance.

QUICK TIP: If a motorcycle has Traction Control, it also has ABS. But just because a motorcycle has ABS doesn't mean it has Traction Control.

Here's where it gets a little confusing. There's another piece of electronics called *Electronic Stability Control* (ESC) that helps you ride even more safely. Stability Control combines ABS, Traction

Control, integrated brakes, and lean angle sensors into one system.

When the system senses that an *out-of-control stat*e is imminent (slide-out, over-acceleration, rear tire lock-up, etc.), it applies one or both brakes (and/or reduces engine power) to keep the bike stable.

ESC is like Traction Control on steroids.

Traction Control for MotoGP

MotoGP racers have experimented with Traction Control systems with mixed results. Some like it. Some don't. When asked what he thought about Traction Control, MotoGP champion Valentino Rossi said:

> *"Having the Traction Control system makes riding the motorcycle much easier, and allows me to open the throttle more rapidly without launching me into a highside. Unfortunately, it takes away from the rider's natural ability and feel for the*

motorcycle, and makes it easier for people to compete with those who they couldn't before having this rider aide. It is basically cheating."[1]

At some point in the future, I predict we will all be riding motorcycles with Stability Control. When this happens, the naysayers—the same riders who don't have a clue what triggers lowside and highside crashes—will still be moaning that they don't need any electronic aids on their motorcycles.

In the end, it's your choice. Choose wisely.

QUICK TIP: It's important to remember that ABS, Traction Control, and Stability Control can't overcome the laws of physics. If you ride outside the limits of available friction, you will lose control. But most motorcycle crashes could have been avoided well within these limits. Remember what my motorcycle mentor used to tell me. TRUST YOUR TIRES.

RIDE A MOTORCYCLE WITH TRACTION CONTROL or STABILITY CONTROL (both include ABS) ... and say goodbye to most single-vehicle lowside and highside crashes.

Key Points

1. Traction Control prevents your rear tire from spinning when accelerating by reducing engine power.
2. Some riders will never embrace electronic aids on their motorcycle. Bad call.
3. ABS, Traction Control, and ESC can't overcome physics, but they can certainly reduce your chances of crashing—and that's good enough.

THIRTY-FIVE

Misinformation on Braking

Now that we have the head knowledge of how ABS, Traction Control, and Stability Control can keep us safer, let's talk about *braking*.

Warning: There's probably more misinformation on how to CORRECTLY USE YOUR BRAKES than on any other topic.

The forums are the worst. I just spent thirty minutes looking online for how to properly use motorcycle brakes, and every forum thread I read was plastered with incorrect information. In each forum, the most incorrect posters were the loudest and crudest.

It's hard to argue with an idiot who thinks he's right.

THIRTY-SIX

Use Your Front Brake

Stay in the habit of using the front brake every time you brake, even if your machine has integrated front/rear brakes or anti-lock brakes.
— David L. Hough

NOTE: This chapter is for normal motorcycles—the ones designed by engineers. If you ride a homemade chopper, skip ahead because the physics here probably doesn't apply. *Do choppers even have front brakes?*

The first thing to know about motorcycle braking is that you should mostly USE YOUR FRONT BRAKE. Rider coaches know this, but somehow some riders don't.

A ton of test data shows that 70 to 90 percent of a bike's stopping power comes from the front tire (front brake). This is because weight is transferred to the front of the motorcycle when you apply your brakes. When this happens, the front tire has more stopping power (friction), and the back tire has less.

Pure physics.

HERE'S the SIMPLE TRUTH. IF YOU ONLY use your rear brake, it's going to take you LONGER TO STOP than me. EVERY–SINGLE–TIME.

It's the same way on a car. The front tires provide the vast majority of the stopping power. Have you ever driven with your emergency brake engaged (by accident) and hardly noticed it? That's because most emergency brakes on automobiles only engage the rear brakes.

Cruiser Magazine said it best:

> *"Hopefully, deliberate avoidance of the front brake [only using the rear brake] is limited to a few dinosaurs (who are likely to be extinct rather quickly). The don't-use-the-front-brake concept shares one thing with all those other [misguided] braking theories: it's wrong."*[1]

Key Points

1. USE YOUR FRONT BRAKE.
2. During emergency stops, the rear brake does very little.
3. If you mostly use your rear brake, change your habit.

THIRTY-SEVEN

How Much Rear Brake?

The rear brake is one of the most misused controls on a motorcycle, which is why it's important to better understand its benefits in different situations.

— *Sport Rider* Magazine

Most experts generally agree that you should predominantly use your front brake. From there, things get a little muddy.

Some suggest that you use a small amount of rear brake, and some suggest that the situation dictates how much rear brake to use—if any.

There's one school of thought that says you're better off using your front brake exclusively during emergency stops because the back tire gets so light and prone to lock up. We all know by now that a locked-up rear tire usually leads to a lowside or highside crash, right?

Just checking.

Before you turn up your nose at the idea of using your front brake exclusively, consider what one thought-leader in the riding community thinks. Keith Code, one of the best known and most successful on-track motorcycle instructors in the world, said:

"The obvious mathematics of the situation is that the front wheel can do 100 percent of the braking and the back, at that point, just locks up no matter who you are. Learn to totally rely on the front brake for quick, clean stopping; then, if you still have a use for the rear, go ahead and use it. But realize that the rear brake is the source of a huge number of crashes, both on and off the track. I'll leave the final decision up to you. While it is true that a motorcycle will come to a full stop quicker with both brakes applied, in racing, you don't come to a full stop until you're done."[1]

Keith knows what he's talking about, yet he gets blasted in online forums for his position on braking. I just spent an hour reading rude insults in three different forums. It frustrates me that so many riders think they know more about braking than Keith.

Note to the guy on the [undisclosed] forum. Keith is not the idiot; *you are*.

And the fact that you think you know more about braking than he does proves it.

More Test Data

An engineering firm, Mechanical Forensics Engineering Services LLC, conducted tests on several different motorcycles to measure the effectiveness of front and rear brakes. Tests results showed:[2]

USING THE FRONT BRAKE BY ITSELF DELIVERED SIMILAR DECELERATION G-LOADS AS USING BOTH FRONT AND REAR BRAKES TOGETHER.

The study concluded: “A motorcycle’s rear brake contributes very little (or even nothing) to the overall stopping power when efficient use is made of the front brake.”[3]

James Davis, an expert witness in Motorcycle Dynamics, said:

> *"Since you can generate nearly 100 percent of your stopping power with the front brake on almost any contemporary motorcycle (meaning that you can reduce traction of the rear wheel to zero via load shifting), there is a pretty strong argument that can be made that you should focus your entire braking attention to the task of using it [your front brake] and ignoring the fact that you even have a rear brake. I would not go that far, however, [because] the use of both brakes together will invariably slow you down more quickly than using just one of them."*[4]

NOTE: Before we go any further, it's important to make this point. Most experts agree that it's best to use *both* brakes when it's been raining, or the road is slippery. This is because less weight is transferred to the front tire when there's less friction to stop you. ABS really helps here.

The Bottom Line

Studies have shown that adding rear brake can help you stop about ten percent more quickly than using your front brake by itself.

But ... USING YOUR REAR BRAKE ALSO SIGNIFICANTLY INCREASES THE CHANCES YOU'LL CRASH.

Not because you hit the object you're trying to avoid, but because

—you lock up your rear tire and lowside or highside on your own!

WARNING: You might want to sit down before you read what I have to say next. It's going to shock some of you, but it's a point I have to make.

I believe that FEWER RIDERS would CRASH AND DIE every year if the REAR BRAKE was REMOVED on all street MOTORCYCLES.

Don't misunderstand me. I'm not advocating this.

I'm simply making the point that your rear brake is one of the most dangerous controls on your motorcycle.

Proficient braking habits begin with this head knowledge.

So, how much rear brake should you use?

If you have ABS, you're probably better off using *both brakes*.

If you don't have ABS, you're probably better off concentrating on using the *front brake* effectively.

Whether you add some rear brake is your decision.

Whatever you decide ...

PREDOMINATELY USE YOUR FRONT BRAKE!

Key Points

1. While experts don't agree on exactly how much rear brake you should use, they do agree that you should use significantly more front brake than rear brake.
2. If your motorcycle has ABS, apply both brakes.
3. Don't dismiss your rear brake yet. Using your rear brake in low-speed maneuvers can provide added stability and control. More on this in a future *Motorcycle Smarts* book.

THIRTY-EIGHT

The Hurt Report

We can reduce our risks by studying how other riders have crashed.
— David Mixson

Now that we understand how electronics can help us keep from crashing, let's take a look at a study that shows us why motorcyclists crash. The *Hurt Report* is considered by many to be one of the most comprehensive studies of motorcycle accidents ever conducted.

I read it when I started riding, and it changed everything.

Background

The NHTSA selected the University of Southern California (USC) to conduct the study entitled: *Motorcycle Accident Cause Factors and Identification of Countermeasures Volume 1: Technical Report.*[1]

The USC professor leading the study was Harry Hurt, Jr. Since the study's official title was such a mouthful, it quickly became known as the *Hurt Report*. Thank goodness.

The purpose of the Hurt Report was to determine the causes of motorcycle accidents, to analyze the effectiveness of protective gear, and to determine what riders could do to keep from crashing.

Professor Hurt's team studied every motorcycle accident in a two-year period (900+) in the Los Angeles Basin area in Southern California. The team collected data from the scene of each accident, reviewed police reports, and interviewed eyewitnesses—including the rider if he survived the crash.

Still Relevant?

A lot has changed since the Hurt Report was published back in 1981. Motorcycle tires and brakes are much better (good things), but roads seem more congested, and drivers seem more distracted (bad things).

Journalist David Hough interviewed Hurt in 1999 and asked him if he thought his study was still relevant. Hurt said:

> *"The more time that goes by, the less things look different. Riders today have the same sort of accidents as riders in the 1970s—except that today they crash much more expensive bikes."*[2]

Hurt also said this during the interview:

> *"I still do consulting for police departments and have investigated a number of police motorcycle accidents over the years. Police*

motor officers get some extensive training. I mean really good training. But even professionals make the same sort of mistakes as novices, and today's riders seem to have the same sort of accidents as those in the NHTSA [Hurt] report."[3]

Numerous NHTSA studies, published since the Hurt Report was released, continue to show similar findings.

Riders are making the SAME MISTAKES that they did nearly 40 YEARS AGO. Think about how UTTERLY INSANE this is. It's one of the main reasons I WROTE THIS BOOK. I wanted to present the information that I think is MOST IMPORTANT in a way readers could understand—a different way—the way I wanted to learn when I started riding.

From all my studies, I believe that Hurt was right.

Riders are still crashing because they aren't using their front brake; because they don't understand what happens when they lock up their rear tire; and because they don't know what do when they start going wide in a turn.

Becoming a proficient rider begins with head knowledge.

The Hurt Report is packed with useful information.

The Hurt Report reveals WHY RIDERS CRASH. It highlights the most common rider errors and shows us how to avoid the most common types of crashes.
POWERFUL STUFF.

If you're serious about changing your chances of crashing, reading and understanding the Hurt Report (and acting on the data in it) is one of the best things you can do. We'll take a deeper look at some key points in the next two chapters.

I read the Hurt Report before I bought my first motorcycle. It gave me confidence that I could reduce my chances of crashing.

It can change your chances of crashing too.

Harry Hurt passed away in 2009. He was 81.

THIRTY-NINE

Hurt Report Golden Nuggets

If you rush through the next two chapters, you're missing some of the most powerful points in this entire book.
— David Mixson

The Hurt Report isn't just a bunch of numbers. It shows us what we should focus on to reduce our risks.[1] It's more than 400 pages.

No worries. I'm going to pull out ten of the best nuggets (five in this chapter and five in the next chapter) and explain how we can use the information to ride safer.

Before we dive in, I want to congratulate you on making it this far.

I realize some of the information in this book wasn't easy to get through, but you've done it.

Thank you for sticking with me.

You're in the home stretch.

Here are five of my favorite golden nuggets in the Hurt Report.

Hurt Report Golden Nugget #1

Hurt found that 25 percent of motorcycle accidents were single-vehicle crashes (motorcycle *did not* hit another vehicle) and that 75 percent were multi-vehicle crashes (motorcycle *did* hit another vehicle).

In addition to this, a 2009 NHTSA study found that 46 percent of all motorcycle fatalities occurred in single-vehicle crashes.

MY THOUGHTS:

When both data points are analyzed, we find that a fourth of all crashes were single-vehicle crashes, yet almost half of the fatalities were in single-vehicle crashes. This means half of the deaths were in a fourth of the accidents—when riders crashed by themselves.

It also means that if you crash all by yourself, you're more likely to die than if you're hit by another vehicle.

Surprising, but useful.

What causes single-vehicle crashes? Keep reading.

Hurt Report Golden Nugget #2

Hurt found that rider error accounted for 67 percent of single-vehicle crashes. Typical errors were:

(1) locking up rear tire and lowsiding, and

(2) running wide in a curve due to excess speed or under-cornering (not using enough countersteering to tighten the turn).

Other causes were animals, blowouts, and surface hazards.

Hurt also found that rider error accounted for about 33 percent of multi-vehicle crashes and that most multi-vehicle crashes were caused when the motorist violated the motorcyclist's right-of-way.

MY THOUGHTS:

Two-thirds of single-vehicle crashes and one-third of multi-vehicle crashes were due to rider error. This doesn't surprise me. I have seen a ton of videos on YouTube where the rider went wide in a turn (because he didn't use countersteering to tighten his turn) or locked up his rear tire and lowsided (because he didn't use his brakes properly).

Using the numbers above (along with basic math), I calculated that 17 percent of all motorcycle crashes were single-vehicle crashes caused by rider error, and 26 percent of all motorcycle crashes were multi-vehicle crashes caused by rider error.

THIS MEANS THAT 43 PERCENT (ALMOST HALF) OF THE ACCIDENTS STUDIED IN THE HURT REPORT WERE CAUSED BY RIDER ERROR.

There's another point worth considering. How many of the accidents determined to be the motorist's fault in the Hurt Report could have been avoided if the rider would have known how to control his motorcycle more proficiently?

Probably a lot.

To all the riders who say, "I can't change my chances of crashing," I say nonsense. You CAN reduce your risks of being in an accident by improving your offensive and defensive riding skills.

The Hurt Report proves it.

Hurt Report Golden Nugget #3

Hurt found that nearly 28 percent of multi-vehicle crashes involved an automobile turning left in front of (or into) a motorcyclist.

My Thoughts:

Every rider should know this tendency so they can know to look out for it. If you could take this crash scenario off the table, you would be less likely to crash on a motorcycle. Even if you could only cut your chances in half of being hit by a motorist turning left in front of you, you would meaningfully reduce your chances of being in an accident.

This statistic was a huge motivator for me when I started riding—and it continues to be something I look out for every moment I'm on a motorcycle. I scan ahead, anticipate when automobiles approaching me might be turning left across my lane, and adjust my position so I won't be in their path if they do.

Hurt Report Golden Nugget #4

Hurt found that motorists failing to recognize and detect motorcycles was the leading cause of accidents.

My Thoughts:

Reading this changed the way I ride. Now, I assume motorists have a hard time seeing me and judging my speed and distance. Be visible, install running lights, wear bright gear, and don't ride at night.

It's your responsibility to be seen.

Have you ever pulled out in front of a motorcycle when you were driving an automobile? I have many times, not because I have a thing against motorcycles, but because I didn't see them or misjudged their speed. I'm betting you have too.

Hurt Report Golden Nugget #5

Hurt found that most accidents were close to the trip's origin (usually home) and involved running an errand or meeting with friends.

My Thoughts:

Never let your guard down. Always ride with the correct gear and the proper mindset—regardless of whether you're one mile from home or a thousand miles from home.

The Hurt Report is packed with useful information that gives us clear clues on how we can ride more safely. I'll highlight five more in the next chapter.

Key Points

1. Don't be the idiot who says you can't reduce your risks. The Hurt Report proves that we can change our chances of crashing—and it shows us how.
2. Don't crash by yourself. Watch out for motorists turning across your lane. Be visible and assume motorists can't see you. Take every ride seriously—even ones close to home.

FORTY

More Hurt Report Golden Nuggets

I hope your mind is racing with ideas on how you might implement what you've learned so far from the Hurt Report.

I know mine was when I first read it.

Here are five more golden nuggets in the Hurt Report.

Hurt Report Golden Nugget #6

Hurt found that riders didn't make the correct evasive maneuver to avoid crashing in most cases. Even worse, riders didn't attempt *any* evasive maneuver 32 percent of the time.

In addition, Hurt found that braking errors were frequently made during the collision-avoidance maneuver when riders attempted one. Riders overused their rear brake and locked up the rear tire (leading to a lowside), and underused (or failed to use) their front brake (leading to longer stopping distances).

Hurt said:

> *"Skidding from over-braking was the most common execution problem, and usually resulted in a loss of control of the motorcycle. Failure to use the front brake is a critical element in collision avoidance because proper use of the front brake would have avoided many of the collisions or greatly reduced the severity. [In most accidents] the ability to countersteer and swerve was essentially absent. In other words, riders didn't stop the correct way and didn't swerve to avoid the crash."*[1]

In Hough's interview back in 1999, he asked Hurt if riders should practice evasive maneuvers. Hurt responded:

"Use the front brake."

"Use the front brake."

"Use the front brake."[2]

MY THOUGHTS:

Frankly, every time I read this finding I get mad. This one piece of information from the Hurt Report puts everything in perspective and reveals just how unskilled some riders actually are. One-third of riders didn't know enough (well enough) to even attempt to stop or make their motorcycle go in a different direction to avoid a crash.

Maybe it would be easier if I didn't care so much.

Riders are missing the fundamentals.

Don't skid your rear tire. Understand countersteering with your head, then practice using it to control your bike until it becomes a part of your muscle memory.

Why? So you can do *something* to avoid a crash. Understand what causes lowside and highside crashes so you can avoid them.

USE YOUR FRONT BRAKE.

Come on riding community. Learn enough about controlling your motorcycle so you can do something to dodge a crash. Don't just sit there like 32 percent of the riders Hurt studied.

When Something Is Coming Your Way

While we're talking about the subject, let's quickly go over what you *should* do if you're about to hit something: (1) look where you want to go (away from the object your trying to avoid), (2) apply your front brake to reduce your speed, and (3) use countersteering to swerve away from the object and toward an opening or a less dangerous object.

If you can do these things, you might be able to avoid crashing (or at least make the crash less severe).

If it sounds like I'm starting to repeat myself, you're getting it.

What you've learned in this book is the foundation of how to control your motorcycle when you're just PUTZING AROUND in your neighborhood. It's also the foundation of how to control your motorcycle when you want to DODGE A CAR spinning out of control towards you. It's the same.

Hurt was an avid motorcycle rider for most of his life and continued educating riders well after the Hurt Report was published. I find it powerful that he never stopped asking riders to use their front brake.

I believe USE-YOUR-FRONT-BRAKE is the first rule of braking because Professor Hurt told us so.

Hurt Report Golden Nugget #7

Hurt found that chest and head trauma were the leading causes of death and that the use of a motorcycle helmet was the single most important factor in the prevention or reduction of head injury.

My Thoughts:

I'll let you draw your own conclusions on the relevance of wearing a helmet and protective gear. They do what they're designed to do.

I wear both.

Hurt Report Golden Nugget #8

Hurt found that riders who took hands-on training from professionals were the *least* likely to be in an accident and that motorcyclists taught by friends and family were the *most* likely to be in an accident.

My Thoughts:

Don't ask your cousin to teach you how to ride a motorcycle. Take hands-on training from professionals.

Hurt Report Golden Nugget #9

Hurt found that riders between 16 and 24 years old were significantly *overrepresented* in crashes and that riders between the ages of 30 and 50 were significantly *underrepresented*.

MY THOUGHTS:

Don't let your age dictate your emotions. I won't let my 18-year-old son ride a motorcycle, and I don't apologize for it. Now you know one of the reasons why.

Hurt Report Golden Nugget #10

Hurt found that nearly half of all riders killed in motorcycle crashes were under the influence of alcohol.

MY THOUGHTS:

If you ride your motorcycle to a bar to get wasted, you're an *idiot*. I don't have a softer way of putting it. I also recognize that absolutely zero riders who do this have made it to this point of the book.

I know—I'm preaching to the choir on this one.

Key Points

1. According to the Hurt Report, riders are missing the fundamentals. Don't lock up your rear tire. Understand and use countersteering to control your motorcycle. Do SOMETHING (brake, countersteer) when you're about to crash. Wear a helmet if you want to protect your head in a crash. Don't rely on a friend to teach you how to ride. Don't drink and ride. USE YOUR FRONT BRAKE.
2. Share some of your favorite Hurt Report takeaways with your riding buddies.

FORTY-ONE

Target Fixation

Look where you want to go because that's where you're going.
— DAVID MIXSON

No book about motorcycle control would be complete without at least a short discussion of the topic of this chapter. Studies have shown (and I've proven it to myself with experiments) that your motorcycle goes where you're looking. It's kind of freaky how this works, but it does.

The phenomena is called *target fixation*. Understanding it can help you avoid a crash if you know how to use it. It can also kill you if you fall victim to its energy.

The key point here is to *look where you want to go*. Sometimes this is easy. Other times it takes extreme focus to make yourself look away from an approaching hazard. Your eyes will naturally fixate on the car sliding out of control toward you, or the huge pothole 20 yards ahead, or the rabbit that decided to stop in the middle of your lane.

When you see a hazard in the road, pick a spot that misses it and look that way. If a car is coming toward you, pick a path that misses the car and look in that direction. Then use countersteering to make your motorcycle follow your eyes.

This sounds so simple, but it can be so difficult.

Try It for Yourself

When you're riding with no traffic or hazards, pick a spot in the road ahead and look at it. Notice how your motorcycle hits the spot. It's amazing. Your body naturally steers the motorcycle in the direction you're looking.

Now you know why it's important to LOOK FAR INTO TURNS when riding around curves. I struggled with this when I first started riding, but with practice it became natural.

Key Points

1. Your motorcycle goes where your eyes tell it to go.
2. Do NOT look at hazards you want to avoid.
3. DO look far into turns in the direction you want to ride.

Nearly Half of all Motorcycle Fatalities are Caused by Rider Error

Part Six: Wrap-Up

In this section, I'll wrap things up and introduce you to *The Motorcycle Smarts*

Creed. You're awesome for making it to this point!

Honestly, this might be the best tip in this book.
Go to the link below and subscribe now.
The book can wait.

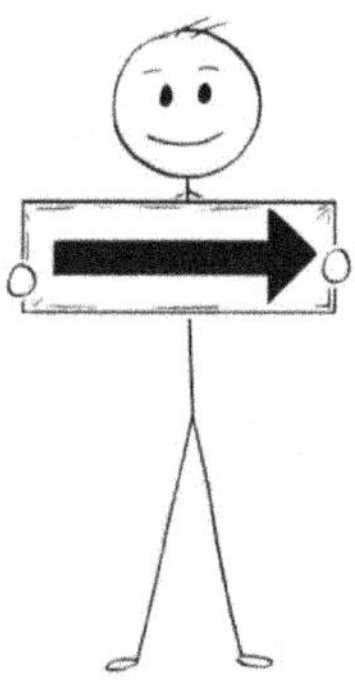

"Motorcycle Smarts"
Quick Tips Newsletter

Free weekly riding tips you can consume in less than 3 minutes—delivered to your inbox for you to use and share with others.

motorcyclesmarts.com/tips

You're not doing everything you can to keep from crashing until you're signed up.

Sign up at the link below.
Unsubscribe at any time.
motorcyclesmarts.com/tips

FORTY-TWO

The Motorcycle Smarts Creed

I wrote this to help me get into the right mindset before I ride.

It's called the *Motorcycle Smarts Creed*.

I will only ride my motorcycle on this day if my mind is clear, my body is rested, and my soul is undistracted.

Today, I will focus on improving my riding skills. I will practice doing what I do well and what I don't do as well.

don't do so well.

I will ride defensively and assume others don't see me. I will watch closely for distracted drivers and give them extra space.

I will position myself so others can see me and ride at a comfortable pace, even if this means I arrive at my destination a few minutes late.

I will represent the motorcycling community to the best of my abilities. I will wave to every motorcyclist, regardless of what they're riding.

I will stay focused on the tasks before me. I will remain patient and expect nothing from the drivers around me. If someone does something stupid, I will not blow a fuse, make a hand gesture, or yell inside my helmet.

I will notice the beauty of nature around me. I will appreciate the smells of changing seasons and the uniqueness of every cloud. I will enjoy the warmth of

the sun shining on me, and the
different shades of green
Mother Nature has painted for
me.
And when my ride is done, and
my thoughts are clear, I will
document today in my journal—
the good, the bad, and the
silent thoughts that pop into my
head only when I ride.
Because today is a special day.

FORTY-THREE

Final Thoughts

When I set out to write this book, I was motivated by the data in the Hurt Report to do something to help riders understand the basics of *how motorcycles work* and *why riders crash.*

Several NHTSA studies have shown that almost half all motorcycle fatalities occurred in single-vehicle crashes—when the rider crashed all by themself. The data doesn't lie.

WE'RE KILLING OURSELVES IN SINGLE-VEHICLE CRASHES BY REFUSING TO UNDERSTAND HOW MOTORCYCLES WORK AND WHY THEY CRASH.

In some ways, it would be more comfortable to blame the distracted driver who pulled out in front of us or the drunken driver who lost control and swerved into our lane.

But that's only a fraction of what's causing us to crash.

THE GUY IN THE MIRROR IS THE ONE WE SHOULD REALLY WATCH OUT FOR.

One of the main goals during my first riding season was to avoid being in a single-vehicle accident. I figured I could at least control this. I was also motivated because the last thing I wanted to do was have to tell my mentors I crashed all by myself.

I remembered this commitment every time I put on my helmet and every time I approached a high-speed curve—the skill I struggled with most in the beginning. I practiced the things I wasn't good at.

I studied what I didn't understand.

I asked my mentors for advice when something felt wrong.

Am I suggesting we can reduce our risks to zero? NO!

Skilled riders crash and die every day when there was nothing they could have done to prevent (or avoid) it.

BUT IT'S ALSO TRUE THAT UNDER-SKILLED RIDERS CRASH AND DIE EVERY DAY WHEN THERE was SOMETHING THEY COULD HAVE DONE TO AVOID IT.

In the end, I believe far too many riders cruise around with a better understanding of what looks cool than an understanding of how to effectively control their motorcycle.

This book was my attempt to change that.

It took me ten years to complete it. I did everything I could to put it off. But I knew deep in my soul that I had to finish it, and I did.

If it helps one rider, I've accomplished what I set out to do when I told my mentors, *"Someday, I want to explain motorcycles my way."*

MASTERING THE ART OF RIDING A MOTORCYCLE WELL is about learning how to ride the right way. It's about taking each ride seriously. It's about enjoying the experience and making good decisions based on the laws of physics.

It's about being confident you can avoid distracted drivers.

It's about having a plan before you need a plan. It takes effort.

It's about understanding and overcoming rider fear, and having the head knowledge of how your motorcycle works so you can make it go where you want it to go.

It's about knowing how to control a motorcycle.

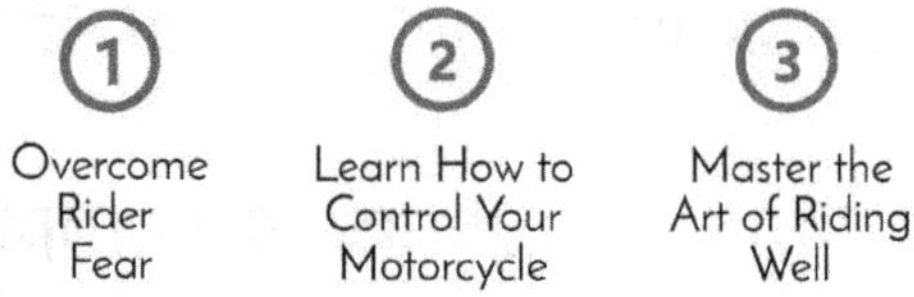
1
Overcome Rider Fear
2
Learn How to Control Your Motorcycle
3
Master the Art of Riding Well

Learning how to control a motorcycle should be your first goal when you buy your first motorcycle, or your next goal if you've ridden for decades. *Control* is the skill that makes you less likely to be in an accident. It's the path to proficient riding.

I honestly believe the information in this book could save your life. But only if you do something with it.

As I said in the beginning:

I believe that riding a motorcycle well is part skill, part willing to learn, part understanding of basic physics, and part giving a damn about your safety and the safety of those around you. THE BALL IS IN YOUR COURT.

Final Challenge

As our time together draws to an end, I leave you with one final challenge to BE INTENTIONAL.

Be intentional about learning how motorcycles work and how to control them, intentional about recognizing and overcoming rider fear, intentional about improving your offensive and defensive riding skills.

Don't be the rider who says you can't reduce your risks. Don't be the rider who doesn't know what the Hurt Report is, what countersteering does, or why you should never lock up your rear tire. Don't be the rider who doesn't wear a helmet because his riding buddies think helmets aren't cool.

Instead ...

Take the information given in this book and use it on your journey to MASTERING THE ART OF RIDING WELL. Practice your craft often.

Take each ride seriously. Learn something new every time you ride.

Keep a journal. Document what you did well and what you need to work on for the next ride. Find a motorcycle that fits your body and your riding goals.

Be wary of drivers turning left across your lane. Riders die every day because of this. Assume motorists don't see you because sometimes they don't—especially if you're wearing dull colors.

And if you're wearing dull colors, ask yourself why?

Know how to use countersteering to put your motorcycle exactly where you want it—regardless of how small you are and how large it is. Consider a motorcycle equipped with ABS and

Traction Control (or ESC) because the advantages far outweigh the disadvantages.

DON'T LOCK UP YOUR REAR TIRE BECAUSE BAD THINGS HAPPEN WHEN YOU DO!

Leave margin so you aren't pressured to ride faster than you want to. Practice in all weather conditions so you'll be ready in real life. And don't be the guy who brags, "My motorcycle has never seen the rain." If you can say this, you've missed out on one of the most memorable things you can do on a motorcycle.

Take a ride to nowhere just because you can. Explore roads near your home you've never been on. Take the long way to familiar places. Discover your city, your state, and your country.

I promise they'll look different on a motorcycle.

Believe you can reduce your chances of crashing because you can.

Use rider fear as a motivator to improve your riding skills or as a sign you should choose a different craft.

Know what to do when you start going wide in a turn and how to keep from lowsiding and highsiding.

USE YOUR FRONT BRAKE! USE YOUR FRONT BRAKE! USE YOUR FRONT BRAKE!

And lastly, represent the sport by being courteous to motorists, choose your riding friends carefully, and embrace the reality that rider safety is a choice—because anyone who tells you different is a liar!

MASTERING THE ART OF RIDING A MOTORCYCLE WELL is a journey, not a destination. Ask any rider who's been doing this for decades, and they'll tell you the same thing—they never stop learning.

I learn something new every time I ride. That's one of the best things about motorcycles—there's always something left to learn, something left to experience, something left to discover. I'm convinced

I'll never have it all figured out, and that's the way I want it.

In the basement of my house back in 2007, I pulled out a perfectly typed set of notes ten pages long and placed it in front of my motorcycle mentors. With more confidence than I deserved, I proclaimed:

"Someday, I'm going to explain motorcycles my way."

In my wildest imagination, I had no idea I would end up here.

I've accomplished what I promised my mentors I would do.

I'VE EXPLAINED MOTORCYCLES MY WAY.

In a deeply personal way, writing these final words feels amazing.

"I finished what I started" feels pretty darn good.

Thank you again for following along and reading what I had to say about a subject I'm so passionate about. I sincerely hope you found something that makes you a better, safer rider. — *David*

FORTY-FOUR

UPDATE: A Case for Mandatory ABS

In the first publication of this book, I was afraid to be so bold.

But this is too important to sit by and do nothing.

By now, you know that I'm a huge proponent of ABS.

So much so that I think ABS should be federally mandated on all street motorcycles sold in the United States. There. I said it.

My hope is that it's already happened by the time you read this.

But just in case. Here's why.

ABS stops most riders more quickly than conventional brakes. But that's not the point I'm going to focus on because that's debatable and has lots of naysayers.

What's even more important to understand is that ABS keeps you from locking up your rear tire and triggering a rider-induced lowside or highside crash—every single time—even when you panic and apply both brakes as hard as you can.

I wrote the *Motorcycle Smarts* book series, in large part, to explain this so all riders and politicians can understand.

It's one of the most important points in this book.

Let me say it a different way.

I WOULD STILL CHOOSE TO RIDE A MOTORCYCLE WITH ABS EVEN IF IT MEANT IT TOOK ME A FEW FEET longer TO STOP THAN RIDERS WITH CONVENTIONAL BRAKES!

The physics explains all this with clarity.

There's no doubt in my mind that ABS would reduce the number of single-vehicle motorcycle crashes. There's no doubt in my mind ABS would lower the overall number of motorcycle fatalities.

Why is this point avoided in other motorcycle skills books?

I believe many riders don't see the need for ABS because their training didn't show them. And neither have the popular motorcycle skills books. If they had, I promise I wouldn't have felt the calling to write the *Motorcycle Smarts* series.

And neither have many of the federally funded crash studies.

The engineer in me says there must be huge opposition to mandatory ABS, or it would already be in place—like it is in Europe. But for the life of me, I can't imagine a viable argument against it.

This is why I explained lowside and highside crashes my way.

Could somebody please show Congress my explanations?

I'm sure folks argued against mandatory ABS for automobiles and light trucks too. But you found a way to pass that legislation.

It's time to do the same courtesy for motorcycle owners.

And while you're mandating ABS, why not go ahead and mandate ESC at the same time? The technology already exists.

If you have ABS and ESC (or Traction Control), you won't be able to spin your rear tire even if you give her too much throttle—further reducing the chances of triggering a lowside or highside crash.

At some point, maybe before you even read this book, I believe ABS *will* be mandatory. At that point, the purpose of this chapter is to convince riders that ABS, ESC, and Traction Control are good.

I know I won't be able to convince all of you.

I just spent my morning looking online at motorcycle forums, and there are certainly some passionate folks against ABS.

Maybe some of the same riders whose bike has never seen the rain?

If the naysayers would look past the stopping distance argument and instead focus on the fact that ABS prevents rider-induced lowside and highside crashes, I think some might reconsider.

If I convert one ABS naysayer, this book series was worth it.

In the first printing of this book, I stopped short of recommending mandatory ABS. After studying the data for my third book, "Motorcycle Hacks," I changed my mind.

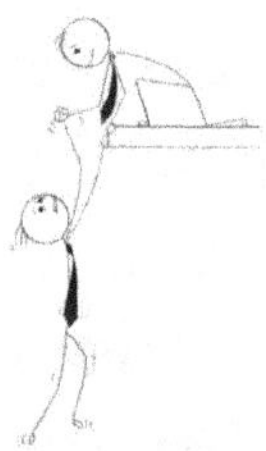

Today. I'm asking Congress to pass legislation that requires ABS (and Stability Control) on all street motorcycles sold in the U.S.

You did this for cars in 2012. Are motorcyclists less important?

Europe passed ABS legislation years ago. It's time we do the same.

If you want to keep everyone happy, make it so riders can manually deactivate ABS when they want to—even though most never will.

I understand that if riders demanded ABS, manufacturers would already be providing it. That's not happening because no one seems to be talking about ABS preventing riders from triggering crashes.

The passionate arguments against ABS focus on stopping distances and the rider having full control (pop a testosterone pill, beat on chest) of his motorcycle without electronics getting in his way.

Give me a break.

FORTY-FIVE

How Can I Help?

My goal in writing the *Motorcycle Smarts* series was never financial.

I'm passionate about the sport, and I hope it shows. If someone wants to champion mandatory ABS on all street motorcycles, I'd be happy to do what I can to help.

I'm also open to sharing parts of the unique content I wrote about in my books with online and print publications—especially the parts about lowside and highside crashes.

Thanks again for following along. —
David

david@motorcyclesmarts.com
linkedin.com/in/david-mixson/

FORTY-SIX

Courtesy Copies for Rider Coaches

My vision has always been to share this book with as many riders as possible. That's my best shot at changing the crash data.

I'd like to start by sending a free copy of this book to as many rider coaches as I can. My hope is that every coach might find a nugget of useful information that they can share with their students—possibly on the topic of what triggers lowside and highside crashes.

Just a suggestion.

But I don't want to stop there.

If I can get enough company sponsorships and individual support, I'd like to provide free/discounted copies to riding clubs and rallies.

Learn more about the *Motorcycle Smarts Dream Team* below.

I can't do this alone.

motorcyclesmarts.com/dreamteam

Appendix

In this final section, I'll introduce my mentors, tell you what folks are saying about the *Motorcycle Mentor Podcast,* and give you a sneak peek of my other books in the *Motorcycle Smarts* series.

Meet My Motorcycle Mentors

I was lucky. I found two men willing to help me when I started riding. Their guidance was less about how to ride the correct way and more about the mental steps you must take to become a proficient rider.

Let's meet them.

Fred Applegate

Fred and I worked together at NASA in the late '90s training astronauts for Spacelab flights and controlling science experiments onboard the Space Shuttle.

Fred retired when he was still young and in good health. With his free time, he played golf, took tennis lessons, and continued enjoying his lifelong passion for riding his Honda ST1100.

Fred is very methodical, detail-oriented, disciplined, cautious, and patient. When I started toying with the idea of buying a motorcycle, I immediately approached him for guidance.

Fred agreed to become my motorcycle mentor.

He graciously helped me through every new challenge. Instead of giving me the answer to my problem, he always guided me toward the solution—knowing that it would have more meaning if I figured it out for myself. Fred was the perfect mentor.

Pete Tamblyn

Pete is one of the top motorcycle instructors in the country.

If you've taken a Stayin' Safe Advanced Motorcycle Training class, Pete might have been your instructor. Over the years, Pete has helped thousands of riders as an instructor at several different riding schools.

Lucky for me, Pete and Fred were roommates back in college and good friends today. Fred refers to Pete as *his* motorcycle mentor. Pete was gracious with his time and always answered my toughest questions with patience and thoroughness.

Thank you both for investing in me, for being patient, for having the heart of a teacher, for encouraging me to follow my passion to start a website, and for helping me write content for the site during the early days. Thank you for helping me ride more safely.

This world needs more MENTORS LIKE YOU!

CPSIA information can be obtained
at www.ICGtesting.com
Printed in the USA
LVHW051636200423
744807LV00010B/330

9 781806 311750